THE CURE

THE CURE

How Capitalism Can Save American Health Care

Dr. David Gratzer

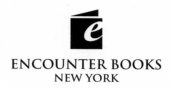

ENCOUNTER BOOKS
NEW YORK

First edition published in 2006 by Encounter Books, an activity of Encounter for Culture and Education, Inc., a nonprofit, tax exempt corporation.

Encounter Books website address: www.encounterbooks.com

"Medicare by the Numbers" is reprinted with permission of the *Washington Post* (© 2006).

The Doctor, by Sir Samuel Luke Fildes, is reprinted on page 11 with permission of the Tate Gallery.

Manufactured in the United States and printed on acid-free paper. The paper used in this publication meets the minimum requirements of ANSI/NISO Z39.48-1992 (R 1997)*(Permanence of Paper).*

FIRST EDITION

Library of Congress Cataloging-in-Publication Data

Gratzer, David
    The Cure: How Capitalism Can Save American Health Care
    / David Gratzer
        p.   cm.
        ISBN 1-59403-153-3
        1. Medical economics.   2. Medical care—Cost control.
    3. Capitalism.   I. Title.
    RA410.53.G73 2006
    338.4'73621—dc22   2006021278

10   9   8   7   6   5   4   3   2   1

To My Family

Contents

Foreword

MEDICAL SCIENCE AND THE PROVISION of medical care were both very different in the United States before World War II than they are now. Before the discovery of the curative power of penicillin in 1941, medical science was able to diagnose disease and to provide care and comfort, but had little to offer in the way of cures. Since 1941, there has been a veritable explosion in medical science that has transformed the practice of medicine. Previously incurable diseases have become curable, pain has become more manageable, general health has improved, and the expected duration of life has lengthened significantly. All in all, penicillin ushered in an age of medical miracles.

Medical care has clearly benefited from these miracles, but in addition it has been revolutionized by developments completely unrelated to medical science. Before World War II, medical care was dispensed through a relatively free market, like other consumer goods and services. The government played a role through the licensing of physicians but was not deeply involved in other ways. The essence of the process was the consensual relationship between the patient and the physician. The patient was free to choose his physician and the physician free to accept or reject the patient. The physician set the fee for his service and the patient paid the fee. No third party was involved in the strictly voluntary transaction between them. Medical insurance covered catastrophic events, not everyday care.

These arrangements were revolutionized by the unantici-
pated effect of wartime price and wage controls imposed to
counter inflation. As always, controls led to shortages—in this
case, a shortage of workers. In response, employers offered
inducements such as "free" medical care. This turned out to be
a particularly attractive add-on and became common. Initially,
employers did not report to the IRS the cost of the medical care
as part of the workers' wages. In time, that practice was legalized
and medical care provided by the employer was made tax-exempt.
Other medical care provided as before, through a direct relationship between a patient and a physician, was not tax-exempt. The
result was that most of the population adopted employer-
provided medical care.

In this way, tax exemption inadvertently changed the provision of medical care from a market, bottom-up system to a
bureaucratic, top-down system. The patient is still free to choose
a physician, though often the choice is subject to severe limits;
but in most cases the patient no longer regards a physician who
serves him or her as "his" or "her" physician, responsible primarily to the patient. Similarly, the physician in most cases no longer
regards him- or herself as primarily responsible to the patient.
He or she will be paid not by the patient but by an insurance company or government official who will have to approve the medical treatment that the physician recommends. The insurance
company or the government is effectively the physician's
employer, and it is their interests, not the patient's, that he or
she is committed to serving.

Exempting employer-provided medical care from taxation
led to the replacement of a consensual system, consistent with
the rest of the economy, by a bureaucratic, third-person payment
system completely inconsistent with the rest of an open economy. The end result has been exploding costs and bureaucratization, as well as widespread dissatisfaction with the system on
the part of both patients and providers.

It is tempting to regard the developments in medical practice as the direct consequence of the developments in medical
science, the high cost and bureaucratization of practice reflecting for the most part the high cost of the drugs, machines, and

procedures that are the product of medical science. This view is a fallacy. Medical science and medical practice are closely related, but the latter is not the consequence of the former, as Dr. David Gratzer demonstrates in this splendid book.

David Gratzer is a practicing psychiatrist who combines firsthand knowledge of medical practice in both his native Canada and the United States with an independent point of view and a rare capacity for lucid exposition of complex technical material. He presents a fascinating and thorough explanation of the developments in medical science and medical practice.

Dr. Gratzer supplements his account of medical science and medical care with detailed and precise recommendations for reform. He gives his recommendations on several levels. For the most part, they accept as given the basic structure of the system, the transformation from a free-market system to a bureaucratic system. However, in his final chapter, "The Three Keys," he proposes major changes that would bring medical care back to a consensual form, restoring it to a system that is compatible with the basic values of a free-market, free-enterprise society.

If you want a well-written, interesting yet authoritative and thorough account of what is wrong with medicine today and how to cure American health care, this is the book for you.

Milton Friedman
Hoover Institution
May 24, 2006

Introduction

IT WAS THE BEST OF American medicine. It was the worst of American health care.

In 2003, when my wife ruptured a disc in her spine, I set about to find her a neurosurgeon in western New York. Uninsured and uninformed, I resorted to cold-calling neurologists, asking for their opinions of reputable surgeons. Few were willing to speak to a stranger about a colleague's skills. Meanwhile, having a choice of two hospitals and no information on either, we selected one at random and then spent a nervous night before the operation at a Hampton Inn, which I had chosen after reviewing detailed reports at Hotels.com. I found myself musing darkly that for a mundane accommodation decision, we had a surplus of data, whereas for a critical medical decision, we had little or nothing to go on.

The surgery itself required only an inch-long incision, took under half an hour, and resulted in an inscrutable bill for an extraordinary sum. When we called to inquire, a hospital administrator hinted that the bill was "negotiable." Before we could negotiate, however, we started to receive threatening letters from a collection agency.

Everyone I know has a story like this, spotlighting something wrong with American health care. The confusion, the paucity of information, the meaningless but always rising prices—all these problems cry out for reform. In response, many policymakers have begun to reconsider the merits of what Hillary Clinton proposed more than a dozen years ago: a publicly managed and financed system of universal coverage—"Canadian-style health care." The CEOs of some private health-care corporations and even some physicians are attracted to the idea.

Not me.

IN MEDICAL SCHOOL, I LEARNED my most important lesson not in a classroom but on the way to one. On a cold Canadian morning about a decade ago, late for a class, I cut through a hospital emergency room and came upon dozens of people on stretchers— waiting, moaning, begging for treatment. Some elderly patients had waited for up to five days in corridors before being admitted to beds. They smelled of urine and sweat. As I navigated past the bodies, I began to question everything I thought I knew about health care—not only in Canada, but also in the United States. Though I didn't know it then, I had begun a journey into the heart of one of the great policy disasters of modern times.

Like most Canadians, I believed that we had the best-run health-care system in the world. Because the system was publicly owned, I assumed that compassion came before profit and that everyone got good care. Sure, there were problems: people sometimes waited to see specialists or to get certain tests. But I didn't know of anyone who died waiting for care, and it seemed especially clear to me that this system was better than America's, with its uneven quality and absurdly high cost.

These views didn't rise from deep philosophical beliefs. I absorbed them from my environment, much as I did my love of hockey. If all politics is local, the corollary is that all policy is personal; and because my family and I were in good health, I didn't see health-care policy as relevant to my life. Politics and policy were not my passions. I wanted to be a doctor.

After I entered medical school, however, my view of Canadian health care changed. The more I was exposed to the system, the more familiar I became with the shortcomings of government-run health care. I trained in emergency rooms that were chronically, chaotically, dangerously overcrowded, not only in my hometown of Winnipeg, but all across Canada. I met a middle-aged man with sleep problems who was booked for an appointment with a specialist three years later; a man with pain following a simple hernia repair who was referred to a pain clinic with a two-year wait list; a woman with breast cancer who was asked to wait four more months before starting the lifesaving radiation therapy. According to the government's own statistics, some 1.2 million Canadians couldn't get a family doctor. In some rural areas, town councils resorted to lotteries: the winners would get appointments with the only general practitioners around.

As pervasive as these problems were, they were accompanied by an equally pervasive public silence. Canadian politicians and voters alike endorsed the status quo. No one, it seemed, wanted to rock the boat. I believed that Canadians deserved better, and I decided to write a book about what I saw and knew.

I had a simple thesis: To contain costs, governments restricted the supply of health care. As a result, while politicians might dismiss waiting lists as a minor inconvenience, the reality was that patients suffered and, in some cases, died. The only solution, I concluded, was to move away from government command-and-control structures. To emphasize the gravity of the situation, I titled my book *Code Blue,* the term used when a patient's heart stops and hospital staff must leap into action to save him.

The book caused a stir. Through call-ins on radio shows and questions asked at town hall meetings, I found that a surprisingly large number of Canadians realized there were significant problems with their health-care system; and increasingly, these problems were reported by the media. Shortly after *Code Blue* was published in 1999, a young man died of an asthma attack because the overcrowded emergency room at his local hospital had not been accepting patients. A chorus of voices were soon criticizing Canadian health care, culminating in 2005, when the Supreme Court of Canada ruled that a law banning private insurance conflicted with the citizen's right to life. The justices reasoned: "The evidence in this case shows that delays in the public health-care system are widespread, and that, in some serious cases, *patients die* as a result of waiting lists for public health care" (emphasis added).[1]

Yet even as public opinion and reform efforts in Canada were moving toward more privatization, in the United States they have been moving in exactly the opposite direction. As I am licensed to practice in both countries and have worked in both, I have been unsettled to see mistakes made north of the 49th parallel repeated to the south. Granted, there are profound differences between Canadian and American health care. But the direction of American health reform—toward greater government intervention—is eerily familiar. It's like watching a car accident unfold in front of me: a series of small events, leading to a spectacularly disastrous end.

THE PROBLEM AND THE PREDICAMENT of American health care can be stated in a single, paradoxical sentence: Everyone agrees that it's the best in the world, but nobody really likes it.

On the one hand, we are so blessed with medical breakthroughs that we take them virtually for granted. Cardiac care has been revolutionized in only a few short years; death due to cardiac disease has fallen by nearly two-thirds in the past five decades. Polio is confined to the history books. Childhood leukemia, once a death sentence, is almost always curable. Depression and other mental illnesses are treatable. Americans are at the forefront of this medical revolution; people from all over the world seek American medicine when they need help. And American excellence isn't confined to the hospital: When three hundred leading internists were asked to rank major medical innovations in a survey for the journal *Health Affairs,* eight of the top ten they ranked were developed, in whole or in part, in the United States.[2]

Yet while the quality of American *medicine* has never been better, angst over American *health care* has never been greater. The state of Medicare, the cost of prescription drugs, and the numbers of uninsured are all considered crises. In a Market Strategies poll, 86 percent of respondents expressed deep concern about rising costs. Six out of ten regarded the likelihood of bankruptcy due to major illness as a serious problem.

Why is American health care such a mess? This book attempts to answer that question. In the process of writing it, I visited five countries and two dozen states, interviewing hundreds of people. As varied and complex as the problems were, I found that they all flowed from a simple, central truth: While the rest of the economy has moved forward, American health care is stuck in an outmoded economic model, dating back to the Second World War.

IN CHAPTER ONE, I OBSERVE that modern medicine began six decades ago with the first clinical use of penicillin. In the following years, medical miracles have been discovered in quick succession. The health of Dick Cheney symbolizes the progress of medicine: despite four heart attacks, he can function in the second-highest office in the government. But if medicine can do more than ever before—literally changing our understanding of life and death—the cost has spiraled upward as well. Adjusting for inflation, Cheney's pacemaker costs more than fifty times the average annual health-care expenditure of an American in 1950.

As I relate in Chapter Two, American health care is an accidental system, arising largely from a fluke tax ruling in World War II. When the IRS announced in 1943 that employer-sponsored health insurance would not be taxed, many employers began offering insurance to their employees as a way around wartime wage controls. While the wage controls were repealed at war's end, the tax exemption has remained. The burden of providing health care—unlike other basic needs such as food, clothing, or shelter—would continue to fall on employers and, later, on government. This burden has increased as medicine itself has become more sophisticated and expensive. In fact, the hegemony of the insurance model has coincided almost exactly with the era of modern medicine. These two forces, the insurance model and technological advances, are mutually reinforcing: because insured patients don't pay directly for their own state-of-the-art care, they can't make the consumer choices that would curb the cost of this high-end treatment. As costs have increased to the point of crisis, reformers have sought to reduce them.

In Chapter Three, I argue that four decades of reforms have failed because they have been premised on two bad ideas—one favored by Democrats, the other by Republicans, and both worsening the problems they were intended to solve. The first alternative was formulated by Wilbur Mills, who championed the creation of Medicare and Medicaid when he was chairman of the House Ways and Means Committee. The second alternative was introduced by President Richard Nixon, who hoped for cost control through HMOs. While both men retired amid scandal in 1974, their competing visions are still doing damage, like the opposing blades of a scissor. Because of the need to constrain rising costs, government programs have led to rationing and price controls. Because of its restrictions on patient choice, managed care has outraged American sensibilities. Consequently, both visions have now lost their luster. America's health-care policy predicament is now akin to Eastern Europe's political *terra incognita* after the collapse of the Berlin Wall: Everyone knows what doesn't work, but no one knows how to proceed. The crisis will only deepen until we find a third way between the Scylla of big government and the Charybdis of bureaucratic HMOs.

In Chapter Four, I map a route between these two hazardous extremes. I explain that both failed options share one fatal feature: they remove choices from patients and give them to government or corporate bureaucrats. Restricting patient choices in this way, flouting the laws of basic economics, has been a mistake. It's the reason why, while pocket calculators have declined in price from $500 to $5, the price of pacemakers keeps rising. If governments free the health-care sector to innovate, we can see price decline in health care, though maybe not to the same degree as in electronics. Consumer-driven heath care offers a promising mechanism to facilitate this. I therefore propose to move choices back to people, so that health care can be improved by the same principles that reward consumers in every other economic sector. In the chapters that follow, I consider how patient choice can be used to insure the uninsured, provide cheaper prescription drugs, and even save Medicaid and Medicare.

In Chapter Five, I focus on the plight of uninsured Americans. While the uninsured reportedly number 46 million, I show that, in fact, 93 percent of Americans either are insured or have ready access to insurance. Government efforts to help the remaining 7 percent are deeply misguided. For much of the past decade, initiatives to cover the uninsured have been straight out of Wilbur Mills' playbook—massive expansions of Medicaid and heavy regulation of insurance. By requiring insurance companies to cover more procedures, for instance, New Jersey has priced even the most basic coverage beyond the reach of the working poor (a family policy costs more than the lease of a Ferrari). To truly help those without coverage, Congress should take two steps. First, it can reduce the cost of health insurance by creating a national market for it, allowing people to opt out of expensive state regulations. Second, the $40 billion of federal hospital grants and other programs aimed at uninsured Americans should be turned over to state governments, which should be allowed to experiment with voucher systems for private insurance.

Interstate experimentation can be used not just to insure more Americans, but also to help those covered by Medicaid, as I explain in Chapter Six. Like so many other parts of the current system, Medicaid insulates recipients from the consequences of their actions, since it almost completely lacks a basic deductible or copay. This program is bureaucratic and expensive, and it fails to get the desired results—in other words, it's much like the old welfare program. Therein lies the best clue to a solution. Just as Congress reformed welfare in the 1990s, so too can it devolve Medicaid to the states. This will encourage innovation, since the temptation for states now is to avoid sweeping reforms (Washington, after all, picks up most of Medicaid's expenditures). States, in turn, can decentralize decision making to recipients. In Colorado, for example, the severely disabled poor can choose a program that empowers them with heath dollars; participants are able to hire and fire their own caregivers, and to use moneys for life-enhancing equipment. Widespread innovation has been stifled, however, by Washington's micromanagement.

If federal meddling has thwarted reform of Medicaid, it has brought Medicare to the brink of disaster, as I show in Chapter Seven. Cost outlays for Medicare are projected to consume one-third of all federal income tax by 2030. This looming financial reckoning has been generated not just by the aging of our population, but by structural problems in the program itself. Medicare covers many small bills, with almost no deductibles or copays, yet it leaves the elderly exposed to potentially enormous out-of-pocket expenses for catastrophic events. Medicare is so inadequate that most seniors carry supplementary insurance. These issues should be addressed by allowing seniors to choose better insurance to begin with—and the Federal Employees Health Benefits Program (FEHBP) offers a perfect model. It is the nation's most successful health plan, and it works because it offers federal employees a choice from more than 240 competing plans. As a result, it contains costs better than Medicare, though it typically covers more things—long-term care, catastrophic events, and even the item that is now so controversial: prescription drugs.

Chapter Eight narrows in on the prescription-drug conundrum. Although prescription drugs do more for us than ever before, the pharmaceutical industry has never been more demonized. Both in and out of Washington, many debate the misguided idea of reimporting prescription drugs as a way of saving consumers and governments money. Yet if reimportation is the wrong prescription, there are nevertheless problems with the current drug regime. Between hungry trial lawyers and meek FDA bureaucrats, the cost of developing a prescription drug is much higher than it needs to be, and new drugs take too long to get to market. With a handful of simple reforms, however, Washington could cut approval times and the cost of pharmaceuticals—and make them safer too. By incorporating safety measures that are readily implemented with information technology, a recalibrated FDA could speed drug approval with a competitive system of certification, and then monitor the approved drugs.

In Chapter Nine, I return to the scene of my original health-care epiphanies and explore some lessons to be learned from health policy outside the United States. Despite the proven economic benefits of competition and choice, many pundits would junk the present system of public and private insurance, and replace it with a Canadian- or European-style system of universal public coverage. As single-payer proponents love to claim, these systems "cost less" overall, provide modern health care, and do so for every single citizen. But these "compassionate" systems can't escape basic health economics, and they end up rationing care in the most draconian ways. For that very reason, once-socialized systems in countries from Britain to Sweden are embracing market reforms. But if single-payer proponents lack practicality, they do have imagination. American policymakers, too, ought to think big.

In the concluding chapter of the book, I set forth my own three-part vision for revolutionary change. First, I argue that America needs to make health care truly individual and portable. Whereas employer-sponsored health insurance made sense in the days of the company town, health coverage should not be tied to employment; rather, people should be enabled to purchase their own coverage (perhaps through their church or union) by changes in the tax code and trimming of regulations. Second, I propose to downsize the FDA and return it to its original mission—judging a drug's safety. A de-emphasis on "efficacy" would streamline the incredibly complex and laborious approval process in which almost a billion dollars is needed to bring a drug to market; this would allow pharmaceutical innovation to flourish and would drive down the cost of new drugs. Finally, I argue that Washington should shore up Medicare, in part by allowing today's workers to save for the health expenses of their elderly years. This will give baby boomers more choice— and leave more money in the Treasury, too. These three bold ideas, combined with the other reform proposals I have developed here, can make American health care better, cheaper, and more accessible for everyone.

In today's political environment, these ideas may seem unrealistic. But then again, conceiving of a future without polio would have seemed equally farfetched just a short time ago. America is a great nation capable of great things. We've seen this time and again in the advances of modern medicine. We can see it with health care as well.

What follows in these pages is a comprehensive look at American health care that points the way to a better system, and avoids the nightmare scenarios I have seen in Canada. Americans should never be forced into the hell of Canadian-style waiting lists. But there must be an alternative to the purgatory of rising costs and uneven quality. The way out is to embrace the policy solutions used to improve every other aspect of the economy— that is, to recognize that innovation and choice can exist only when we unleash the forces of capitalism.

ONE

Dick Cheney's Heart

Medicine's role is to entertain us while Nature takes its course.
—Voltaire

IT ISN'T BEAUTIFUL, BUT IT is art. Luke Fildes' *The Doctor* is an engraving of a concerned physician watching over a gravely ill child. It is remarkably lifelike, perhaps in part because it is based on Fildes' own experience: his son died before adolescence. The engraving, made in 1887, says much about medical practice at the time. The doctor looks distinguished, deep in thought, and

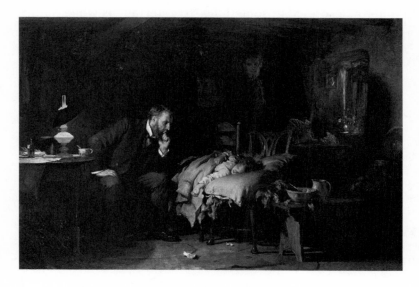

empathetic. In a time of crisis, he is there and ready. But notice what the doctor is not doing—much of anything. He sits in his chair, pensive but immobile. The physician, in fact, isn't doing much more than the distraught father. There are no IV poles or cardiac monitors or oxygen prongs. There is no intervention.

People tend to think of medicine as an ancient tradition. Doctors trace the origins of their profession back to the days of Hippocrates. Organized medicine, too, claims deep roots. The American Medical Association was founded during James Polk's presidency. The American Psychiatric Association claims the revolutionary hero Benjamin Rush as its founder. Historians paint a similar picture. *Timetables of Medicine,* a breathtaking book on the evolution of medical practice, contains only two pages on developments since the mid-twentieth century. But medicine as we know it—a world of powerful antibiotics and MRI scanners—is a thoroughly modern creation.

Fildes' engraving captures the essence of medicine in its time. By the early nineteenth century, doctors had established a battery of treatments: bleeding, purging, complicated diets. By the 1830s, however, many doctors understood that these treatments did more harm than good. As a result, for most of the nineteenth century and the earlier part of the twentieth century, they had little to offer except comfort for the ill. Medicine was as Voltaire described it: something "to entertain us while Nature takes its course." Consider that when Sir William Osler—arguably the most prominent physician of his time—helped found the Johns Hopkins School of Medicine in the late nineteenth century, most drugs available were more harmful than beneficial. Oliver Wendell Holmes commented that there were only five drugs worth saving from the fishes; one of them, incidentally, was mercury.[1] Dr. Osler spent much of his career taking patients off medications.

In *The Rise and Fall of Modern Medicine,* the British physician and columnist James Le Fanu describes the limitations of medical practice around the turn of the century:

> The pattern of human disease had changed little over the previous 2,000 years. The problems of infectious disease—both acute and chronic—dominated medical practice, culling the young

either early in infancy or later from lethal childhood illnesses such as whooping cough and measles. The causes of the diseases that emerged from adolescence onwards—schizophrenia, rheumatoid [arthritis], multiple sclerosis—were unknown and had no specific remedies. Those who survived into old age were vulnerable to chronic degenerative diseases of ageing—cataracts clouded their sight, arthritic hips limited their mobility—and succumbed from age-determined illnesses of the circulatory disorders and cancer.[2]

This state of affairs would change dramatically after 1941, beginning with an experimental treatment for the consequences of an ordinary injury.

A policeman named Albert Alexander scratched his face on a rosebush. The wound grew septic and the resulting infection ravaged his body. His face was studded with abscesses; he lost his left eye; his lungs were filled with fluid. Alexander seemed destined to die in the septic ward of his local hospital. Fortunately, Dr. Charles Fletcher decided to try an entirely new treatment: penicillin. On February 12, 1941, Alexander was given the antibacterial agent. There was so little of it available that his treatment team collected the patient's urine to harvest the penicillin after administration. By day four, Alexander's temperature broke.

Many battles were fought in 1941; this one changed the way we live and die.

It's easy to forget how different the world was before penicillin. Rich and poor could die of infection within one or two days. As president, Calvin Coolidge had access to the best doctors in the country, but it did little good when his son fell ill in 1924. At age sixteen, Calvin Jr. enjoyed tennis on the White House courts. Playing one day without socks, he developed a small blister, which became infected. He died soon after. The president, one of the most powerful people in his time, crawled on all fours in an attempt to catch a rabbit so that his son could hold it while he died. "In his suffering, he was asking me to make him well," remembered Coolidge. "I could not."[3]

Penicillin has spared countless other parents from such heartbreaking helplessness. It has proven to be such an important discovery that even if no further breakthroughs had occurred in the twentieth century, we could still rightly consider it the Century of Medicine. But penicillin was just the first in a long string of medical miracles. Dr. Le Fanu lists nine more breakthroughs in *The Rise and Fall of Modern Medicine,* and dozens more could easily be named. What is striking is how recent all these innovations are: not a single item on the list was developed before 1941. In other words, most of the best years of Ted Williams' baseball career predate a large part of modern medicine.

Ten Defining Moments for Modern Medicine
(according to Dr. James Le Fanu)

1941	Penicillin
1949	Cortisone
1950	Smoking identified as a cause of lung cancer
	Tuberculosis cured with streptomycin and PAS
1952	Chlorpromazine in the treatment of schizophrenia
1955	Open-heart surgery
1963	Kidney transplantation
1964	Prevention of strokes
1971	Cure of childhood cancers
1978	First test-tube baby
1984	Helicobacter identified as the cause of peptic ulcer

Before 1941, many great improvements were made in public health, allowing people to live longer and healthier. Few of these changes had much to do with the practice of medicine; they involved better housing and nutrition, safe water, and (to a lesser extent) improved hygiene. Once people got sick, however, doctors weren't much help: except for a few treatments such as thyroid hormone, insulin, and bone setting, patients got better pretty much on their own. Or they didn't.

But look at the changes in the latter half of the twentieth century. Doctors now had drugs to use: antibiotics, steroids, lithium. Surgery progressed immensely, with the help of antibiotics and anesthesia. Doctors no longer merely offered comfort; instead, they were busy curing patients. Today, those who have followed in the footsteps of Sir William Osler can prescribe more than five sister drugs related to Prozac alone. CT scanners have been bested by MRI scanners, which are now outdone by PET scanners. Surgery helps everything from sick hearts and worn hips to fetal abnormalities—correcting problems even before birth.

Dr. Le Fanu cites examples of the profound results. Every single child who contracted leukemia in 1950 died; today almost all survive. Children with congenital heart disease or kidney failure formerly lived as pitiful invalids if they lived at all; now they lead relatively normal lives.

Not everyone has embraced the changes in medicine whole-heartedly. In the late 1970s, the sociologists Darryl Enos and Paul Sultan argued that doctors had given up their mission as comforters of the sick; by way of comparison, they quoted from an article published in the *Journal of the American Medical Association* in 1927: "One of the essential qualities of the clinician is interest in humanity, for the secret of the care of the patient is in caring for the patient."[4] Senator Edward Kennedy complained about the rise of specialists. Sidney Wolfe (of Ralph Nader's Public Citizen group) bemoaned doctors' growing dependence on machines. *Newsweek* argued that medical education was transforming young physicians into "mere technologist[s]." But doctors didn't worry about such complaints: the symbolic physician sitting in Fildes' engraving had gotten out of the chair and started saving lives.

Certainly in my field, psychiatry, it's difficult not to see the benefits. For example, schizophrenia is a mental illness that leaves patients psychotic or perhaps catatonic. In the past, many were warehoused in asylums—beyond the help of society, they were banished from view. In 1950, there was no drug treatment for schizophrenia. Patients were treated with shock therapy (without anesthetic, leaving them with broken bones), insulin comas (which carried a mortality rate of up to 10 percent), and lobotomies. Today, thanks to the new antipsychotic drugs, many patients with schizophrenia can live in the community and avoid symptoms for years at a time. One father who saw his son being salvaged from the shores of insanity told me, "This has meant the world to me."

Consider the major advances of the last three decades. Caroline Poplin lists them in an article for the *Wilson Quarterly:*

The results came in a rush: widespread use of ventilators, the development of intensive care units, and the computer-assisted tomography (CT) scanner, the introduction of cardiac bypass surgery, all in the 1970s; fiber-optic devices and magnetic resonance imagers (MRIs) in the 1980s, which made possible diagnoses that heretofore had required invasive surgery, along with recombinant DNA pharmaceuticals, and materials and techniques for total joint replacement; and, finally, in the 1990s, laproscopic surgeries, which permit surgeons to perform major procedures such as gall bladder removal and chest lymph-node biopsy through a few inch-long slits, thus allowing patients to go home the same day.[5]

In medical circles, it is often remarked that half of all medical treatments in use today were invented in the last quarter century. In fact, even the most common ailments—like depression and hypertension—are treated with medications that didn't exist just two decades ago. And the innovation continues.

It is not just medicine that has been transformed; so have our expectations of life. Star quarterbacks throw touchdowns into their forties. Seniors populate the country club's green— and also the Senate and the Supreme Court. Retirement, once seen as a brief interlude between work and death, spans decades for some. Old age has been redefined. Just thirty years ago, any British citizen who reached his or her hundredth birthday was personally congratulated by the queen. Today, there are so many people joining the centenarians' club in the United Kingdom that civil servants draft the congratulatory notes. A similar trend exists in the United States and across the Western world. Aging is largely a modern phenomenon. When *Hamlet* opened at the Globe in the early days of the seventeenth century, only one in forty people were age 65 or older. Today, about one in seven people in the Western world are 65 or older.

These advances in health and longevity have unquestionably improved our lives—but at what cost?

My Heart Surgery and Dick Cheney's

As a rule, a politician expressing a desire to remain in high office seems about as newsworthy as a district attorney saying that winning cases is better than losing them. So when Vice President Cheney told reporters that—should the president ask him—he would be available to run for re-election, the remark generated little if any press. But it should have been a matter of interest that Cheney felt up to the job. After all, he suffers from severe heart problems. Dick Cheney's health can tell us a great deal about the advances in medicine—and about the problems with today's health care.

Health care has steadily emerged as a major political issue. It was the promise of universal health care that helped the unlikely candidacy of Bill Clinton in 1992; it was the fear of cutbacks in Medicare that hobbled Bob Dole four years later. Health care colors local and national politics in practically every election cycle. Yet health care is a very *modern* political concern. Nowhere in the Declaration of Independence does Thomas Jefferson worry about the British influence on American hospitals; as visionary as the Constitution is, not once does it mention managed care. But understand Cheney's heart and you understand the transformation of American medicine.

Consider that the vice president had suffered four heart attacks, the first when he was just thirty-seven. Several cardiologists have speculated that his heart's ejection fraction—measuring how efficiently the heart is pumping—may be less than half that of a healthy man.

That isn't how we think of the vice president—as a man with half a heart. Dick Cheney is a major player in the White House. Some have suggested that he is the most influential vice president in history. Whether or not that is true, this much we can all agree on: Mr. Cheney is a very busy man. When Iraq became the administration's focus, he went to the Middle East, touring a dozen nations in just ten days. During the midterm election, he became a presence in congressional races from coast to coast, campaigning for more than ninety candidates.

How can Cheney be so tremendously functional with such health afflictions? Since his problems were first discovered, he has had a variety of major interventions. In 1988, for example, doctors performed a heart surgery, bypassing four clogged heart vessels with grafted veins from his leg. When the Florida recount dominated the news after the 2000 election, he had an angioplasty, a procedure in which a tiny balloon was threaded through his heart to the clogged blood vessel, then expanded—literally cracking open the constricted area—and then a small wire mesh, or stent, was placed there to keep the artery open. Finally, in 2001, Cheney received a pacemaker, one with the capacity not only to speed up his heart, but to shock it if the rhythm becomes erratic.

As a society, we have grown so used to rapid medical advances that we tend to forget their magnitude. I'm as guilty of this as anyone, having spent two months in a cardiac surgery rotation in medical school. Six weeks into the rotation, the surgeon invited me to assist right up to the moment when the heart was stopped and the bypass machine was turned on. It was like a movie: I was standing in the OR beside a famous heart surgeon, the bright lights beaming down on me, and the beating heart just beneath my trembling fingers. This was the pinnacle of modern surgery, and what did I feel? Boredom. At the hospital where I trained, three operating theaters pushed through six, sometimes eight heart surgeries a day. I sat through procedure after procedure, with awe and excitement fading to a calm interest and eventually settling into bored indifference. The first bypass surgeons expected that their procedure would remain rare. After all, they reasoned, only a healthy young man could possibly endure the surgery. But today, heart surgery has become routine, and not just for the healthy and young. I was once asked to see a 92-year-old man, post-bypass.

Contrast the situation just six decades ago: Days after the Japanese attacked Pearl Harbor, Prime Minister Winston Churchill came to the United States to help cobble together the wartime coalition. History remembers his stirring speech to Congress and then his equally eloquent address in Ottawa, followed by his portrait session with Yousuf Karsh, resulting in the most famous Churchill photograph. But in the middle of the trip, on December 26, 1941, his personal physician believed that Churchill suffered a heart attack. Dr. Moran considered prescribing the state-of-the-art cardiac care of that time: six weeks of bed rest. Treatment of the underlying pathology was unknown. Fortunately, Churchill carried on, leading Britain through the war.[6]

As much as medicine has advanced since then, it's striking how little it had changed in the previous century. For example, when General Robert E. Lee suffered a heart attack on the battlefield at Fredericksburg in the spring of 1863, the state-of-the-art cardiac care was bed rest for two weeks. This noninterventionist approach left something to be desired. Today, a physician who treated a heart attack with bed rest would lose his license.

Heart attacks are still a common problem, but a much less serious problem than they were just a few years ago. Dr. Nortin Hadler, an internist with the University of North Carolina and a medical consultant to ABC, summarizes the statistics:

> My chance of having a heart attack at sixty is about 50 percent less than my father's chance when he was my age. If my father had suffered his first heart attack when he was my age, his five-year potential for survival would have been about 50%.
>
> If I have a heart attack, my likelihood of living another 5 years is at least 95%.... If I take a baby aspirin from the time of my first heart attack, the likelihood of surviving 5 years rises to better than 97%.[7]

The death rate from heart attack and heart failure has fallen by more than half since 1950, from 307 per 100,000 Americans to 126 in 2000. The long-term effects of a heart attack have also changed. According to the American Heart Association, 88 percent of heart attack survivors under age 65 return to work. The Heart and Stroke Foundation of Canada conducted a major international study of health after a heart attack. Amazingly, they found that 44 percent of American heart attack survivors felt their health was *better* after one year than in the month before the cardiac event.[8] As the *Washington Post* observed, "Americans have heart attacks that are becoming smaller and less lethal.... Although heart attacks remain exceedingly common and serious problems,

Death by Cardiac Disease
per 100,000 Americans

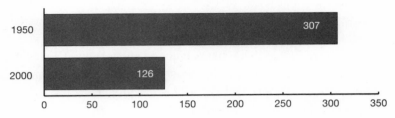

Source: American Heart Association

the data suggest that people's chances of surviving them have increased dramatically."[9]

What accounts for the great increase in survival rates and well-being? Cardiac care has been revolutionized in the last six decades. Part of the innovation lies in drug intervention. Using chemicals found in bacteria, scientists have developed specific drugs that eat away at the source of the heart attack: the clot in the coronary artery. Many patients who have a heart attack are now eligible for thrombolysis, using streptokinase, urokinase, or tPA. Beta-blockers, a class of drugs that slow the heart, given within a few hours of the cardiac event and continued for a year, reduce mortality by about one-third.[10] Other interventions help markedly in reducing the disability caused by heart attacks: bypass surgery, for example, ends the pain of angina. The drugs and procedures that have made so dramatic a difference in the lives of millions of Americans are essentially all new. The quadruple bypass surgery that Mr. Cheney had in the late 1980s dates only from the late 1960s. Angioplasty was developed in the 1980s. Advanced pacemakers are newer still.

But the revolution in medicine has come at a stiff price. The economist John Goodman calculated that if every American went to his family doctor and requested all the blood tests available, it would cost more than the entire GDP of the United States. And Americans are interested in more than blood tests.

Consider the costs of cardiac care. The clot-busting drug tPA costs thousands of dollars per use; heart bypass surgery costs tens of thousands of dollars; the special pacemaker in Mr. Cheney's

chest, known as an ICD or "implantable cardioverter defibrilla-
tor," costs between $20,000 and $25,000. Let's put this figure in
some perspective. The little box in the chest of the vice president
costs more than fifty times what the average American spent on
health care (adjusted for inflation) for an entire year in 1950.[11]

Economists often comment on the rise of health expenditures in the United States, and with good reason from a fiscal
point of view. But noting the growth in spending without considering its results is myopic. Yes, medical expenditures have risen
dramatically, but are the results worth it?

David Cutler has been considering this question for years.
A Harvard professor, he served on President Clinton's Council of
Economic Advisers. In the 1980s, he formed a working group with
fellow economists Mark McClellan (now with the Department of
Health and Human Services), Harvard's Joseph Newhouse, and
Dahlia Remler of Columbia, to study the costs and results of cardiac care. Sitting in his corner office in Harvard's University Hall,
Prof. Cutler explains his calculations. He assumes that for every
year a life is extended, the value is $100,000. "It's a bit arbitrary,"
he concedes.[12] After all, how can you price the priceless? Still,
$100,000 is "mid-range" for most economic analyses. In 1950, there
was almost no spending on cardiovascular disease. Today, the
average 45-year-old will have to shell out $30,000 on cardiac care
in his life. But he will also live longer, by about 4.5 years. Cutler
notes that not all of this increase in lifespan is because of medicine; harmful behaviors like smoking are less common today. He
also makes other adjustments, such as the cost of keeping people alive in nonworking years. Still, he figures that the value added
is about $120,000—a fourfold return on expenditures. By his cal-
culations, furthermore, *all* of the cost increases in medicine over
the past fifty years have been offset by the value of the advances
in just two areas: cardiac care and help for low-birth-weight infants.

We might question Prof. Cutler's basic premises. Why
$100,000 for a year of life? Why not $25,000 or $125,000? To whom
is the year of value? Society? The individual? Are all years created equal—a year of life for a 25-year-old man has the same value
as for an 85-year-old? But in Cutler's defense, it should be pointed
out that others too have come to the conclusion that we get good

value from modern medicine.[13] Maybe attempting to quantify "value" is a mistake when it concerns a life. The father of an ailing low-birth-weight infant, for instance, would not be satisfied with the best medicine of the 1950s for his daughter. Medicine may cost more than ever before, but it also does more than at any time in our history.

David Cutler's work speaks to the changing nature of medicine: it is moving past the days of cures and into a new era of choice. Value is becoming more subjective.

"Save a life—your own!" advertises a New York clinic that offers full-body scans. These scans are the ultimate in preventive medicine: they can diagnose a problem years before a patient becomes symptomatic. Clinics boast of people saved by the diagnostic test: nonsmokers who discover lung tumors; healthy men with early (and treatable) renal carcinoma. Some are unconvinced—including the American College of Radiology, which finds no good argument for scanning healthy individuals.

Full-body scans may be more about hypocondriasis than about hypervigilance, but genetic testing serves a clearer purpose. About one in eight American women will develop breast cancer; the percentage is much higher in those with a family history of the disease. For a price, women can be tested for a gene, BRCA, that is heavily linked to cancer. A positive test, however, is not a sure indication of future cancer. Nor is the information of much practical utility: besides mastectomy, there is no treatment for a breast cancer that has not developed yet.

Diagnostic medicine isn't the only area where the line has been blurred between good medicine and mere personal desire. Pharmaceuticals now target problems that have little to do with extending life. Viagra, the blockbuster drug for erectile dysfunction, is a case in point, as is Rogain, a hair regrowth treatment.

People taking certain types of medications—like cholesterol-lowering drugs—may have some choice of treatment for their underlying problem. Statins, the most commercially successful class of drugs in history, have been shown to do their job and do it well. But in milder cases of hypercholesterolemia, diet and exercise can also lower cholesterol. Many people—such as my ever-busy brother—choose the medication instead. Increasingly, treatment is open to individual preference.

All of this should be the beginning and end of a marvelous story: after centuries of research and discovery with little to show for the efforts, medicine was transformed in a few short decades, improving virtually everything about our lives. Yet if medicine has never been better, Americans have never been so dissatisfied with their health care. This leaves us with a grim and difficult question: Why has the delivery system failed so miserably to match the advances of the products it brings?

Two Days That Changed Health Care

IF THE ERA OF MODERN medicine began with a bang—the discovery of penicillin in 1941—the era of modern American health insurance began with a whimper. The biggest event to shape American health insurance occurred on October 26, 1943, when the Internal Revenue Service issued what seemed at the time like a mundane tax ruling.[1] For the first time, the IRS confirmed that employees were not required to pay tax on health insurance premiums paid on their behalf by their employers. Health benefits would remain tax-free, an idea codified in the new Internal Revenue Code of 1954.

The ruling had its roots in the wage and price controls imposed by the administration of Franklin D. Roosevelt as part of the war effort. "Where any important article becomes scarce, rationing is the democratic, equitable solution," declared President Roosevelt on April 27, 1942. The effects of price control are well remembered—for instance, a black market for gasoline. But wage control also produced a side effect, as employers sought to find ways to provide employees with competitive salaries without violating wage control. Across America, employers found their answer in health benefits. The IRS ruling legitimized the practice, establishing the supremacy of third-party payership and the importance of employer-based coverage.

David Henderson, who served on President Reagan's Council of Economic Advisers as a senior economist for health-care policy, remembers internal discussions within the council as to why so many employees had such lavish health benefits. He explains the attraction of employer-based coverage: "If the marginal tax rate is only 20 percent, then an employer and employee can avoid 20¢ in taxes by shifting $1 from pay into tax-free health insurance. But if the marginal tax rate is 40 percent, shifting that same $1 helps avoid 40¢ in taxes."[2] Henderson observes that throughout the 1950s, 1960s, and 1970s (with one major interruption for the Johnson-Kennedy tax cut of 1964), marginal tax rates kept rising, which made it increasingly attractive for employers to shift compensation from taxable money payments to nontaxable health insurance.

Henderson recounts conversations with Martin Feldstein, the Harvard economist who served as chairman of the Council of Economic Advisers:

> Feldstein gave examples like the following (which I updated with 2000 data): Consider an employer and an employee trying to decide on an extra dollar in taxable wages or an extra dollar of health insurance. The employee is earning, say, $40,000. If this employee has a spouse who earns $25,000, the family is likely to be in the 28% federal tax bracket. The social security tax rate (for employer and employee combined) is 12.4%. The Medicare tax rate (employer plus employee) is 2.9%. The employee's family is likely to be in at least a 5% marginal state income tax bracket. The marginal tax rate of this employee, who is by no means unusual, is 28% + 12.4% + 2.9% + 3.6%,[3] for a whopping total of 46.9%.
>
> Thus, almost *half* of an additional dollar of cash compensation goes to various governments and it is this half that can be avoided by taking additional compensation in health insurance rather than in cash. As long as the employee values an extra $1 in health insurance at more than about 53.1¢ (100 – 46.9) he or she is better off taking it in that form.[4]

There is one problem with low-deductible and low-copayment plans: they cost a great deal to administer. A claim may still cost $20 to process even if it's for a $50 doctor's visit. Why would employees want such a wasteful system? Henderson suggests it's a matter of economics:

The employee is better off to charge a $50 doctor's bill to the insurance company—even if the company spends $20 to process it—and have the employer pay the extra $70 in a higher premium to cover the bill and the processing cost. The alternative—having the employer pay an extra $70 in cash—yields the employee only about $42 and costs the employer $75.36 ($70 + $5.36, the employer's portion of the social security and Medicare tax on $70).[5]

For the employee, then, seeking a job with generous health benefits makes sense, particularly for those in the higher tax brackets. Rather than seeing nearly 50 cents on the income dollar lost to taxes, he or she gets a full dollar of health benefits. For the employer, there is a clear advantage as well: it's more effective to offer lavish health benefits than to raise wages. Both the employer and the employee gain by this arrangement. Before wage and price controls, employer-based health coverage was relatively rare. By 1987, a full 70 percent of employers offered health benefits.[6] So common is employer-based coverage that insurance industry executives refer to the individual policy buyers (that is, people buying coverage for themselves) as the "residual market."

But employers and employees aren't actually getting something for nothing. There *is* a group that supports the whole scheme: taxpayers. Making health benefits tax-free is, in fact, a massive tax subsidy. The so-called tax exclusion amounted to $188.4 billion in 2004.[7]

With regard to the health tax exclusion, then, a few observations. First, when we calculate total government health expenditures to be around 46 percent of all health spending, we underestimate. After all, we haven't considered the indirect effect of the tax exclusion, which would add another 10 percent. Second, and far more troubling, is the fact that the tax exclusion is, in effect, a subsidy for the middle class and the wealthy. Usually, tax subsidies are meant to help the less fortunate; but the health benefits exclusion does the opposite. After all, who gets employer-based coverage? More often an employee of IBM than a single mother working as a part-time waitress. Since the tax subsidy increases as the tax bracket climbs, the mail clerk at IBM gets a smaller subsidy than the CEO. The data bear this out: 26.7 percent of all federal tax expenditures go to families with annual incomes of $100,000 or more, even though this group accounts for only about 14 percent of the population. As for those on the other end of the income spectrum, only 28.4 percent of all tax expenditures will go to families with incomes below $50,000— yet this group contains 57.5 percent of all U.S. families.[8]

Bill Thomas, as chairman of the House Ways and Means Committee, observed that a group of employees are the cheapest group to insure—yet they receive the biggest tax breaks. In contrast, people who have the hardest time obtaining coverage get the smallest tax subsidies. Tax policy regarding employer-provided health coverage has created, in Thomas's view, "the most bizarre red-lining concept ever conceived."[9]

Indirect Federal Subsidy of Private Health Insurance,
by Family Income, in 2004

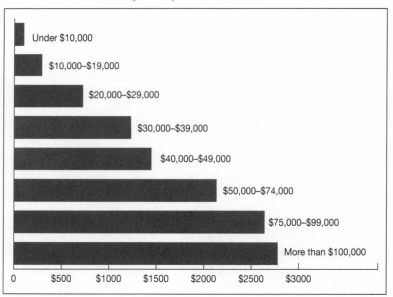

Source: *Health Affairs*

The Beveridge Report

Nonsensical tax policy was not the only concept born during World War II that would profoundly distort the pricing of health care. Around the time of the IRS ruling, Lord William Beveridge released a report to the British House of Commons that would lay the intellectual groundwork for the other dominant force in American health care: the rise of public insurance.

Lord Beveridge had explored the question of how to improve people's lives, concluding that government must take a more active role in providing for the health of citizens. His report, made public on December 1, 1942, served not only as a model for the creation of the British National Health Service, but also as a template for public health insurance in the United States.

Lord Beveridge envisioned a universal public health-care system that was "free." His plan reflected both the paternalism of the time and his own compassion. On the latter point, Lord Douglas Jay, a British MP and intellectual influence of the Labour government of the 1940s, declared:

> Housewives on the whole cannot be trusted to buy all the right things where nutrition and health care are concerned. This is really no more than an extension of the principle according to which the housewife herself would not trust a child of 4 to select the week's purchases. For in the case of nutrition and health, just as in the case of education, the gentleman in White-hall really does know better what is good for people than the people know themselves.[10]

Even aside from the clear misogyny of the comment, it's difficult not to feel that this attitude comes from a different world. In fact, Lord Beveridge *did* live in a different world—a time before the widespread use of penicillin, when life expectancy was far shorter. Stephen Pollard, a senior fellow at the Centre for the New Europe, describes some realities of life in Britain at the time the National Health Service came into being:

> When the NHS was founded in 1948, we Britons lived in a very different country. Food was rationed. Life expectancy was about 50. A third of the houses in Birmingham had no sanitation. Only one in eight married women worked. In working-class, poverty-

stricken Jarrow, infant mortality was 114 per 1,000 births. Even in prosperous Surrey it was 41 per 1,000. Today it is less than 6 per 1,000 for the U.K. as a whole.[11]

At the time, the founding of the National Health Service was considered unimportant. When the *New Statesman,* a center-left publication, reviewed the accomplishments of the Labour government of the 1940s, the essay didn't even mention the public health insurance.[12] But Britons today, whatever their ambivalence about the NHS, look back at the program's creation as a defining moment for their nation. In a poll taken at the end of the 1990s, the establishment of the NHS was ranked as the achievement of the century—polling ahead of, among other successes, winning the Second World War.

Lord Beveridge's report helped legitimize the call for government expansion into health care in the United States (an idea previously weighed down by its Bismarckian, and thus German, inspiration). The British example—and Beveridge's American lecture tour—inspired the American Left. In the 1930s, FDR's staff had debated incorporating health insurance into the Social Security Act but deemed the idea so controversial that it was dropped without any public mention.[13] After the Beveridge Report appeared, FDR declared in his State of the Union address that the social insurance system should extend from "cradle to grave." He openly supported the Wagner-Murray-Dingell bill, which proposed amending the Social Security Act to include health benefits.

That effort failed. But it inspired another, similar initiative, spearheaded by Harry Truman in 1949—which also failed. From the ashes of that grand legislation, however, rose the public programs of the 1960s. As every civics student knows, President Lyndon Johnson flew to Missouri to sign the Medicare bill into law—and to present Truman with the first Medicare card, acknowledging his past efforts.[14] It would have been more appropriate for LBJ to fly to London to mark the event, since the British shadow over American health care is clear. Though American health-care financing is often described as "private" (as opposed to the public systems of Europe and Canada), government plays a major role. Of every dollar spent in the United States, roughly

46 cents comes directly out of local, state, or federal coffers. Even ignoring the tax exclusion, U.S. health care is at least partially socialized.

The bigger influence, though, is structural. The two health programs of LBJ's Great Society—Medicare and Medicaid—are modeled on Lord Beveridge's principles. For the most part, patients don't pay directly for the insured services they receive. Of course, Medicare does include some premiums and coinsurance, but most hospital and physician services require little or no payment from the patient when he or she is treated.

Overinsured in America

December 1, 1942, and October 26, 1943—from these dates flow more than six decades of American health policy. The IRS ruling that addressed wage controls in the days of FDR colors employee health benefits in the days of Google and WebMD. Lord Beveridge's vision of public insurance is now embodied, in the United States, in Medicaid and Medicare. These two defining events have led to the same result: Americans are overinsured.

Because health insurance (both public and private) is all-encompassing—leaving Americans to pay, literally, just pennies on the health-care dollar—we tend to miss the basic point of insurance. Think of car insurance: people purchase it to cover them for accidents and other misadventures. They pay a certain amount of money (the premium) every year in order to avoid a significantly larger expense (such as the cost of fixing a car after an accident) that they have a small chance of incurring. As Lawrence Mirel, the insurance commissioner for the District of Columbia, explains, "An 'insurable event'—from traffic accidents to tornadoes—is something that: first, is very unlikely to happen; second, will come without warning; and third, is not something the person who is insured ever wants to happen."[15] Car insurance—ultimately an insurance against accidents—follows perfectly from Mirel's definition. Contrast this with modern health insurance, in which a large amount of money is paid to cover virtually everything, from major events (cancer) to minor procedures (a yearly physical exam). Car insurance premiums aren't particularly heavy, especially when people purchase high-deductible plans; but the average family's health premium tops $9,000 a year. What would car insurance cost if people insisted on plans that had limited deductibles? Or policies that included not just major body work, but also oil changes and gas and a paint job every time your spouse got tired of the car's color?

Absurdities of this kind are present in health care because health insurance is based on a model appropriate for the conditions of the early 1940s, but not for those of today. Third-party payership reigns supreme. Compared with the astonishing advances in medicine, changes in the structure of health insurance are basically nonexistent. North American visitors to European countries are often struck by the problems of Old World infrastructure; the roads and bridges were built for a different age, when horses and buggies dominated the streets, not Toyotas and Fords. European countries are thus compelled to make a series of unsatisfactory attempts at accommodation: mazes of one-way streets, regulations discouraging the use of large vehicles, sidewalks that substitute for parking lots. In some ways, American health care suffers from a similar malady. We are attempting to provide patients with twenty-first-century care built on an insurance model that hearkens back to the days of FDR and Beveridge. Much of government policy today is an effort to fit the square peg of modern medicine into the round hole of 1940s insurance.

There is a straightforward, if profound, consequence to that effort: health-care inflation.

Why Does Health Care Cost So Much?

Two simple observations can be made about the complex world of American health care:

1. The science of medicine has advanced incredibly over the past sixty years.
2. Health expenditures have grown dramatically over that period.

Most analysts suggest that the advancement of medicine has led to the cost explosion. But is that the right conclusion to draw?

Most would agree that America spends a great deal of money on health care. But as to the merits of that spending, the consensus ends and the debate begins. Some see it as excessive, while others argue that it's not enough. Indeed, there are two positions: the fretters and the spenders.

Fretters worry that the United States spends nearly one-sixth of its GDP on health care; that employee premiums approach $10,000 per year, undercutting corporate profitability and workers' wages; that spending threatens to push state and federal budgets further into the red. "Workplace coverage is becoming unaffordable for many employers and employees," explains Kate Sullivan, director of health-care policy at the United States Chamber of Commerce.[16] (Anxiety-based quotations often come from spokesmen for employer groups—those who foot the bill.)

Spenders argue that health expenditures help people. Americans may have spent less on medicine in the days of President Calvin Coolidge, they argue, but now our children don't die of simple infections. The resulting improvement in our ability to heal has been well worth the added cost. The Princeton economist Uwe Reinhardt predicts that health care will consume 28 percent of GDP by 2030, but asks, "What else would you spend your money on? SUVs?"[17]

Milton Friedman, recipient of the 1976 Nobel Memorial Prize in Economic Sciences, is neither a fretter nor a spender. He thinks both schools are wrong. Health care, he argues, has evolved significantly in recent years. For this reason, however, he thinks it ought to be *cheaper*. That it isn't cheaper suggests to him a major structural problem.

Prof. Friedman has made a career out of dazzling observations. His work on monetary policy (he invented monetarism) helped him land the Nobel Prize and also helped America tame inflation. His ideas have influenced governments from Chile to China. On the occasion of his ninetieth birthday, even Britain's left-leaning *Observer* grudgingly acknowledged that Friedman is the most influential postwar economist in the world.[18] But his health-care hypothesis is not particularly dazzling, because it's based on simply observing every other sector of the economy.

Friedman notes the rapid, nearly dizzying pace of technological advance since the industrial revolution and asks a simple question: Why is it that in every other field where enormous technological strides have been made, total costs have *fallen* over time, but in health care they have increased? "In every other part of the economy," he explains to me in his crowded home office, "growth in an area has been accompanied by declining unit costs and declining percentage of national income."[19]

It was cheaper when I was younger is a comment often heard over the dinner table during holiday meals. Such comments are usually followed by a lengthy list of items that were less expensive only a short time ago. Children who grew up in North America have thus been regaled with tales of stockings that could be had for a quarter and hamburgers that cost a mere 30 cents.

But such comparisons fail to account for inflation. Michael Cox, vice president of the Federal Reserve Bank of Dallas, and Richard Alm, a business writer for the *Dallas Morning News,* argue that price comparisons are deceptive for that reason. In *The Myths of Rich and Poor,* they put forward a better means of comparison: time invested. Cox and Alm reason: "The best way to get around the inflation in money prices lies in figuring what goods and services cost in terms of a standard that doesn't change—hours or minutes of work."[20] In historical comparisons, work time makes far more sense than sticker prices. When stockings could be had for a quarter, the average worker earned 14.8 cents an hour; it would take one hour and 41 minutes of work to buy a pair. Today, stockings require only 18 minutes of work.

Cox and Alm argue that prices have been falling for the vast majority of goods and services, almost always accompanied by a rise in quality. In 1954, for example, a color television delivered a fuzzy picture for a big price: three months of work. Today, the average American worker can get a crystal-clear picture on a 25-inch model for just three days of labor. A bulky calculator in 1972 cost 31 hours of work. Today, a more compact and more powerful one can be had for less time than a leisurely lunch: 46 minutes.

The price of admission for the latest Hollywood offering has fallen from 28 work minutes in 1970 to just 19 minutes in 1997. As for the hamburgers that used to be 30 cents, their real price has fallen, too. The first McDonald's burger had a price of just under 30 minutes of work, but a Big Mac today costs about 8.6 minutes of work and contains more beef.

If most goods and services are getting cheaper, health care in the United States stands as the exception. Consider, for example, the incredible leaps in employer premiums on an annual basis since 1999: 8.2, 10.9, 12.9, 13.9, 11.2, and 9.2 percent.[21] These numbers are particularly striking given that inflation has been so low. We could also take a big-picture view and look at total health spending as a percentage of economic output. Here again, we see a pattern: Americans have never spent more. Milton Friedman provides the numbers:

> Expressed as a fraction of national income, spending on medical care went from 3% of the national income in 1919 to 4.5% in 1946, to 7% in 1965, to a mind-boggling 17% in 1997.

Friedman compares health spending with other sectors of the economy:

> The change in the role of medical care in the U.S. economy is truly breathtaking. To illustrate, in 1946, seven times as much was spent on food, beverages, and tobacco as on medical care; in 1996, 50 years later, more was spent on medical care than on food, beverages, and tobacco. In 1946, twice as much was spent on transportation as on medical care; in 1996, one-and-a-half times as much was spent on medical care as on transportation.[22]

Some would argue that medical care grew more sophisticated over those years. But then, so did the production of food. Today, Americans spend a fraction of what they did half a century ago on food—yet the U.S. agriculture industry feeds more people. In fact, in basically every other area of the economy, the pattern holds. "It's the way we enhance productivity," says Friedman.

Not all kinds of medical care have soared in price. For instance, as cosmetic surgery grows more popular (with network television shows dedicated to the subject), the prices are falling. In 2002, Americans had 1.6 million surgical procedures for cosmetic purposes, a 400 percent increase since 1992; meanwhile, the real prices of these procedures had risen less than inflation.[23] It would be impossible to argue that innovation isn't occurring in cosmetic surgery. While the facelift has been the common method of enhancing appearance, various alternatives now exist: Botox injections, chemical peels, laser resurfacing.

But cosmetic surgery isn't really what we mean by "health care." We tend to think of doctors' offices, MRI scanners, and emergency rooms—and we tend to think of hefty prices. On the whole, advancing medical technology, unlike agriculture or telecommunications, has been accompanied by exploding costs. Why is health care the exception?

The reason is simple: Americans do not pay directly for physicians or hospitals or other health providers A third party makes the vast majority of payments in the United States. And as Prof. Friedman has observed, nobody spends somebody else's money as wisely as he spends his own.

It is true that workers see deductions for health premiums in paycheck after paycheck, causing a frustration great enough to result in, for example, the months-long strike by grocery workers in California. Americans worry about money—a Kaiser Family Foundation poll found that 64 percent of the public is very concerned about not being able to afford the expenses of a family member's illness.[24] But out-of-pocket expenses account for only *14 cents* on every health dollar spent in the United States. Between employer benefits (covering most of working America) and government programs (insuring the poor and the elderly), most of every health-care dollar does not come from individuals (see charts).

For decades, third-party payment has been the standard, so much so that practically every politician today emphasizes the importance of employer-based health coverage. While economists frequently disagree with one another—there's even an old joke that economics is the only field where two people can get a Nobel Prize for saying the opposite thing—health economists time and again use the same phrase to describe America's bizarre arrangement for health financing: it's the "natural order" of affairs.

Health Spending by Source in the United States, 1962, 1982, and 2002

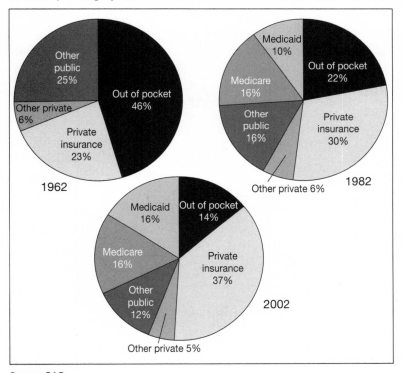

Source: GAO

But there is little that is natural about the arrangement. Consider, for example, the way we pay for food or clothing or housing—all basic needs, just as health care is. Would we expect our boss to keep our fridges stocked with cold cuts and cheese? Did human resources write you a check to cover the building of your family home? Through a regulatory fluke, health insurance fell among an employer's responsibilities. The resulting accidental system is fraught with problems. Imagine how you would shop if you knew that you would have to pay only 14 cents on the dollar of your grocery bill. Nelson Sabatini, formerly Maryland's secretary of Health and Mental Hygiene, suggests that "using health care in this country is like shopping with someone else's credit card."[25]

With such a perverse incentive, it's only a matter of time before someone steps in and attempts to tame costs. Third-party payership, thus, inevitably leads to a bureaucratization of health care. There's an old expression: He who pays the piper calls the tune. With so little being spent directly by the person receiving health care, it is assuredly not the patient who is calling the tune.

Out-of-Pocket Share Falls and Per Capita Spending Climbs

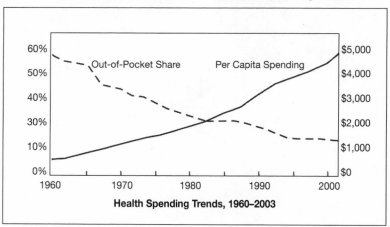

Source: Center for Medicare and Medicaid Services, National Health Expenditures Joint Economic Committee

Bureaucratization has two direct results. First, it undermines patient satisfaction. Despite the incredible advances in medicine, people are frustrated because bureaucrats ultimately decide what gets covered and under which conditions. And it's not just patients who are unhappy. Doctors as a whole are more dissatisfied than ever with the practice of medicine, even though their ability to help a patient with depression or heart disease or dementia is significantly greater than it was thirty years ago. We speak of the high-tech medical revolution; but with health insurance, we have a low-satisfaction era.

The second result is "bureaucratic displacement." Soon after the creation of the National Health Service, the British government was spending significantly more on health care but the system didn't seem any better for it. A physician named Max Gammon sought to solve this policy riddle. After an extensive study of Britain's socialized medicine in the 1960s, Dr. Gammon remarked: "In a bureaucratic system, increase in expenditure will be matched by fall in production. Such systems will act rather like 'black holes,' in the economic universe, simultaneously sucking in resources, and shrinking in terms of 'emitted production.'"[26] His observation applies also to America's partly socialized health-care system today.

For example, several economists, including Milton Friedman, have looked at the input and output of American hospitals.[27] We can measure the output by looking at the number of patient days per 1,000 Americans. Input can be quantified as the cost of providing hospital care for that population. The number of occupied beds per resident of the United States rose from 1929 to 1940 at the rate of 2.4 percent per year; the cost of hospital care per resident, adjusted for inflation, at 5 percent per year; and the cost per patient day, adjusted for inflation, at 2 percent per year.

From 1946 to 1996, the number of hospital beds fell by more than 60 percent; the fraction of beds occupied, by more than 20 percent. In sharp contrast, input skyrocketed. Hospital personnel per occupied bed multiplied ninefold, while cost per patient day, adjusted for inflation, rose an astounding fortyfold, from $30 in 1946 to $1,200 in 1996 (at 1992 prices). The fortyfold increase in the cost per patient day was converted into a thirteenfold increase in hospital cost per resident of the United States by the sharp decline in output. Hospital days per person per year were cut by two-thirds, from three days in 1946 to an average of less than a day by 1996.

Milton Friedman offers an explanation for these trends:

> Taken by itself, the decline in hospital days is evidence of progress in medical science. A healthy population needs less hospitalization, and advances in science and medical technology have reduced the length of hospital stays and increased outpatient surgery. Progress in medical science may well

explain most of the decline in output; it does not explain much, if any, of the rise in input per unit of output. True, medical machines have become more complex. However, in other areas where there has been great technical progress—whether it be agriculture or telephones or steel or automobiles or aviation or, most recently, computers and the Internet—progress has led to a reduction, not an increase, in cost per unit of output. Why is medicine an exception? Gammon's law, not medical miracles, was clearly at work.[28]

This analysis gives a big-picture view of hospital care. Gammon's law seems to plague even the area of medicine that has seen the greatest advances: cardiac care. David Cutler's research (as discussed in Chapter One) indicates that as costs have risen, survival rates have improved dramatically. Jonathan Skinner and his colleagues at Dartmouth extended Cutler's work, looking at the years from 1986 to 2002. Their conclusion: while costs have continued to rise, survival rates have stagnated since 1996.[29]

But shouldn't competition lead to higher standards in medicine, just as it does in other industries?

The Competition Problem

MORE THAN SIXTY YEARS HAVE passed since the IRS ruled that employer-provided health insurance would not be taxed. As I sit in the lunchroom of Pitney Bowes' corporate headquarters in Stamford, Connecticut, the ruling's effect is very much felt. I'm meeting with Dr. Jack Mahoney, a former White House physician who once looked after President Ford. These days, he is looking after a different type of patient: Pitney Bowes, his employer. As corporate medical director, Dr. Mahoney is charged with the task of trying to tame his company's health expenses. Pitney Bowes operates eight medical clinics (logging 31,000 medical appointments a year) and runs a Health Care University that offers courses teaching employees how to use health services better. No wonder, then, that Mahoney and his efforts were profiled in the *Wall Street Journal.*[30]

To Dr. Mahoney, prevention and wellness aren't just buzzwords. The Pitney Bowes head office features its own gym and a doctors' office; there are posters encouraging health on the office walls. "Every patient encounter is a teaching opportunity," enthuses Dr. Brent Pawlecki, the company's associate medical director.[31] He is pleased when patients go to the doctor with a trivial problem like a hangnail. "It means we can talk to them about cholesterol, diabetes, or their obesity." Dr. Mahoney observes that Pitney Bowes spends about 10 percent of its health-care budget on prevention and wellness—roughly five to ten times more than a typical large corporation. But the company's health costs overall continue to climb; Mahoney pegs the annual increase over the past few years at roughly 6 percent, versus 9 percent or higher for other companies.

Why do costs keep rising? Dr. Mahoney mentions ER visits. In cities like Los Angeles and New York, GP offices often close at 5 P.M., so families then seek primary care in emergency rooms. "It's one-stop shopping," he says.[32] Families can get all the tests and consultations needed in one visit when they go to an ER— and not take time off work. That may make sense to families who pay only $75 for the ER trip, compared with $25 for the GP visit. But to Pitney Bowes, the math is much less favorable: roughly $700 for the ER and $75 for the GP.

"Even large companies can't really control costs," says Mahoney. "It's very, very difficult." He remarks that health-care markets just "aren't functional. . . . They aren't transparent to the user. It makes buying an Oriental rug look easy."

Dr. Mahoney isn't a big believer in the magic of competition. If anything, competition seems to be driving health costs *higher.* Diagnostic tests are a major expense for the company; the cost of CT scanning in 2003 was up 7 percent from the year before. Dr. Mahoney believes that the problem lies in the entrepreneurial medical facilities that offer the tests, pushing up costs by offering more services and creating demand. (He recalls seeing a CT scanning facility that offered a two-for-the-price-of-one special.) Doctors' offices have now bought MRI and stress tests. In one study of diagnostic testing in Connecticut, cardiologists who owned such equipment ordered testing four times more often than their colleagues who didn't.[33]

The health industry today appears to teem with competition: drug companies spend billions of dollars on advertising, attempting to convince people to choose one product over its competitors; hospitals work feverishly to attract the interest and contracts of insurance companies; insurance carriers market scores of products to employers, pitting one PPO (preferred provider organization) against another. Yet according to Prof. Michael Porter (Harvard) and Prof. Elizabeth Olmsted Teisberg (University of Virginia), the problem is that American health care lacks the right *type* of competition.

Writing in the *Harvard Business Review,* Porter and Teisberg assess the high-cost, low-satisfaction paradox and conclude that "competition . . . occurs at the wrong level, over the wrong things, in the wrong geographic markets, at the wrong time." Competition, they suggest, should exist at the level of *disease*—that is, the prevention, diagnosis, and management of particular illnesses. Instead, hospitals and health plans at present compete with one another, and the results are higher cost and lower availability.

> Costs are high and rising, despite efforts to reduce them, and these rising costs cannot be explained by improvements in quality. Quite the opposite: Medical services are restricted or rationed, many patients receive care that lags currently accepted procedures or standards, and high rates of preventable error persist. There are wide and inexplicable differences in costs and quality among providers and across geographic areas. Moreover, the differences in quality of care last for long periods because the diffusion of best practices is extraordinarily slow. It takes on average 17 years for the results of clinical trials to become standard clinical practice. Important constituencies in health care view innovation as a problem rather than a crucial driver of success. Taken together, these outcomes are inconceivable in a well-functioning market.[34]

America doesn't really have a market for health *care,* it seems, merely a market for health *insurance* (for third parties).

Journalists sometimes ask campaigning politicians basic questions such as the price of a quart of milk. The results can be embarrassing. When the presidential aspirant Lamar Alexander didn't know the price of milk, he faced a blizzard of critical news stories. There is something to this line of questioning—after all, everyone who goes to a grocery store regularly knows the price of milk. If a politician objects that the inquiry is silly, it can be pointed out that everyone *can* know the price of a quart of milk; the answer is as close as the nearest corner store. But what about the price of a visit to the family doctor or a simple blood test? Walk into a grocery store, and every item has a sticker indicating its price; but have you ever walked into a doctor's office and seen a list of prices? Has it even occurred to you to ask what a procedure or test will cost?

In a normal market, self-interest is useful. The baker, to use Adam Smith's example, isn't getting up at four in the morning because he wants your dinner party to be a success. By the same token, you aren't particularly concerned about your baker's mortgage when you buy a dozen rolls from him. In a normal market, consumers seek good products at attractive prices offered by efficient suppliers.[35] Likewise, producers are always concerned with delivering quality goods and services—and innovating to achieve that goal. The end result is what Cox and Alm describe so eloquently: better products and services at lower prices. But these normal market processes—based on productive self-interest, if you will—have been inverted in the world of health care. In a normal marketplace, people spend their own money. With health care, people spend someone else's money. Although producers in a normal market continuously search for ways to reduce cost, physicians and hospitals face only limited pressure to do so. The success of a physician depends less on service to patients than on meeting requirements of third-party reimbursement formulas. Whereas innovation and technological change in a normal market are viewed as good for consumers, health-care payers are hostile to new technologies because of their high prices.

Herein lies the real tragedy: for all the expense of modern American health care, its quality is suspect. John Wennberg, the director of the Center for Evaluative Clinical Sciences at Dartmouth Medical School, has spent three decades studying regional variations in spending and outcomes. In his recent work, he focuses on Medicare. Many have noted that Medicare spending differs greatly by region, being three times higher in some areas than in others. Thus, an elderly patient in Minneapolis costs $3,341 a year, while a Miami retiree costs almost $8,414.[36] But Dr.

Wennberg and his group push the inquiry further. They find that in some parts of the country, Medicare recipients get up to 60 percent more care than in other areas; yet health outcomes and quality of care are no different—in fact, they are actually *worse* for some types of preventive care. The regional variations aren't explained by gender or race or illness prevalence or the cost of service.

One could fill a book with examples of Americans who were failed by the health-care system. After a car accident, a Florida man was told that physiotherapy would be unnecessary, and he has been left in a wheelchair. A Minnesota man lived under the cloud of depression for years because his family physician didn't understand basic management of the illness. A diabetic from California had a host of specialists, but no one to coordinate the care, meaning that basic preventive measures were not taken.

Everyone knows people who have fared poorly in the murky waters of American health care. But if costs spiral up and quality is suspect, what are employers—or government—to do? One proposed solution has been to increase the management of care, especially through the "health maintenance organization," or HMO. Just as the Founding Fathers studied failed experiments in government, it's worthwhile to study the rise and fall of managed care. In the rubble, we find important lessons.

THREE

Nixon's Revenge

IN 1969, PRESIDENT NIXON USED the word *crisis* in response to a question about health care at a press conference. "We face a crisis in this area," he said. "Unless action is taken in the next 2 or 3 years ... we will have a breakdown in our health care system."[1]

That year, millions of Americans—roughly one in every four households—tuned in to the television program *Marcus Welby, M.D.* Dr. Welby represented everything right about American medicine: he was calm, thoughtful, wise. But if Americans celebrated the successes of the good doctor (and, for that matter, the medical science that made it all possible), they deplored the sorry state of the health-care system he supposedly worked in. *Fortune* magazine ran an issue on medical care, declaring that the system stood "on the brink of chaos." *BusinessWeek* rhapsodized on the cost-effectiveness of European systems, especially as compared with American health care. When a pollster asked heads of families if the system was in crisis, three-quarters agreed.[2] The White House felt that action was needed, so President Nixon offered a new national health strategy in 1971.

For years, Republicans played defense on health care. Government enthusiasts had pushed through initiative after initiative. Washington's role grew larger—paying for hospital construction, funding indigent care programs, and then developing two new entitlements, Medicare and Medicaid. Yet health care remained an issue. In fact, because of these governmental efforts, it became a *central* issue. Medicare and Medicaid threw gasoline on the fire of health inflation. But even though government had helped cause the problem, many saw government as the solution. Governor Nelson Rockefeller of New York proposed a resolution calling for national health insurance, and the National Governors' Conference endorsed it. The Senate Finance Committee mulled a federal takeover of catastrophic insurance. What was the Nixon administration to do?

Nixon embraced HMOs. Previously considered utopian and leftist, health maintenance organizations were now seen as a cost-control tool, which appealed to the president and his aides. But managed care was hardly a stellar success at the time. With fewer than four million members, HMOs appeared to be just a "West Coast thing."[3] Nixon made HMOs the centerpiece of his health strategy and set an ambitious goal: 90 percent of Americans would have the option of enrolling in an HMO within the decade.

And health care would never be the same.

The Rise of HMOs

"The managed care revolution has brought a much more organized, rational way of delivering health care. HMOs and other kinds of managed care companies seek to improve your health status and prevent disease progression, while steering you toward physicians who have better demonstrated quality."—*J. D. Kleinke, health-care analyst and bestselling author of a book on the virtues of managed care, 1996*

HMOs were a new take on an old idea. The concept of managed care actually originated in the fraternal orders and lodges of the late nineteenth century. Many of these organizations had already offered their members life insurance, and health care seemed to be a natural extension. In exchange for an annual fee, physicians provided service. By the early twentieth century, these contracts came under assault from organized medicine. Partly out of blatant self-interest and partly out of genuine concern, physicians fretted over the poor standards of their prepaid colleagues. Some experimentation with prepayment continued (in Washington and Oregon, for example), but the practice faded.

In the late 1930s, the idea gained a new lease on life. Sidney Garfield, a California physician, approached the industrialist Henry Kaiser with an offer. He and his group of physicians would cover Kaiser's Los Angeles construction workers for a set amount, five cents a day. Kaiser accepted. With success in the City of Angels, Kaiser extended the deal to his workers in Washington State. For the employer, prepaid health care offered predictable costs, and physicians felt that patients benefited.

When World War II broke out, Kaiser's shipyards swelled with people—as did the enrollee list for the first large-scale HMO. When the war ended, the shipyards slowed. Kaiser then decided to offer the plan to the public, and the Kaiser health plans were born.

But for decades, HMOs remained a West Coast phenomenon. That changed with Richard Nixon's new health initiative. For Nixon, HMOs represented a two-step strategy: first, he would popularize the idea by making them the standard in employer-sponsored health insurance; then he would turn Medicare over to the HMOs. Thus, the cost-control woes of both private and public insurance would be solved by the HMO gambit.

The White House pushed Congress into action, which resulted in the HMO Act of 1973, an effort to popularize managed care. It had bipartisan support—one of its chief proponents was Senator Ted Kennedy. (So the irony: Nixon's attempt to curb government expansion won the backing of America's foremost advocate of government health care.) To facilitate the startup and expansion of HMOs, the act offered an unusual mix of deregulation and regulation. It overrode state laws that had restricted the development of HMOs, but also required any company with twenty-five or more employees to offer two HMO plans as part of its benefits package. Washington added a remarkable incentive for companies entering the HMO business: $1.6 billion (adjusted for inflation) in grants and loans.

Washington's support for HMOs continued even after Nixon resigned. Pushed by the White House, Congress moved again, amending the HMO Act to further subsidize managed care. Academia, too, warmed to managed care. Alain Enthoven, a Stanford professor (and formerly a deputy assistant secretary of defense under Robert McNamara), argued that increased health spending wasn't always beneficial. Certainly, initial expenses helped a population become healthier (think of basic public health measures and important medications). But after a point, increased expenditures were no longer linked to betterment of health status, he argued. He blamed the problem partly on consumer misuse of health resources, but also on the enthusiasm with which doctors and hospitals pushed treatments (supply-induced demand, to use the technical term). After Enthoven spoke with Paul Ellwood, a businessman and physician, the two became leading proponents of a large-scale effort to manage health care. Ellwood's now-famous vacation home in Jackson Hole, Wyoming, was used to promote the idea to business leaders and politicians.

But while Washington and academia were keen on HMOs, the rest of the country was more hesitant: by the end of the 1970s, total enrollment was only ten million. Nixon's vision seemed to be a failure.

An important factor in the American economy helped push managed care to the tipping point: the continuing rise in health costs. In the mid-1970s, an executive at General Motors noted that BlueCross BlueShield had become a bigger supplier to the company than U.S. Steel. The 1980s saw the problem expand far beyond Detroit. A Robert Wood Johnson Foundation survey in 1988 found that 60 percent of corporate executives labeled health costs a "major concern" and 35 percent called them a "top concern."[4] They were directly invested in the health cost of their employees, and those costs were exploding. The generous benefits that companies had agreed to give their workers were now becoming an overwhelming commitment.

Most Americans had either indemnity plans (insurance companies paid for some of the care), or BlueCross BlueShield policies (the care was provided by their network of doctors and hospitals), or some type of government coverage. For many, deductibles and copayments were minimal; indeed, BlueCross BlueShield policies, by tradition, had neither. As costs exploded, employers began to rethink health insurance; by the 1980s, deductibles and copayments became commonplace (if modest). But employers needed to do more. Within a few years, they would completely revise the way they offered health benefits. In 1988, three-quarters of American workers with employer-sponsored health insurance were covered by traditional (indemnity) plans; by the end of the 1990s, those indemnity plans represented only 14 percent of the market. By 1998, HMO enrollment had soared to 79 million—an eightfold increase in eighteen years.

HMOs went mainstream. In the early 1990s, the insurance giant Aetna wasn't even in the managed-care world; the corporation insured large companies with traditional (indemnity) policies. But when managed care took off, Aetna moved in, embracing HMO policies, expanding into the individual insurance and Medicare markets, and acquiring other firms to increase enrollment. Aetna didn't simply become the largest health plan nationally but also became a dominant player in the most populous regions, including New York, Florida, Texas, and California. Between 1997 and 1999, the number of Americans covered by Aetna jumped from 13.7 million to 21.1 million.

The possibilities seemed endless. In 1995, House Republicans, for instance, under the guidance of the conservative Speaker Newt Gingrich, even suggested that HMOs would help rein in the cost of Medicare. The idea won praise from, among others, Governor Howard Dean of Vermont, who would go on to run for president as the most liberal candidate since Walter Mondale (who, incidentally, served on the board of a Minnesota HMO).

The attraction of managed care in general, and HMOs in particular, was clear. HMOs held down costs with a variety of techniques, such as paying family doctors *not* to refer patients to specialists and utilization reviews of medical practices. To eke out even greater savings, HMOs used their enormous buying power to push hospitals for discounts. For a health-care industry used to the tranquility of indemnity plans—send a bill to the insurance company, get a check back with no questions asked—HMOs represented a perfect storm.

It would take a book to fully weigh the basic strategies of HMOs: selective contracting, innovative incentives, and utilization reviews. The most spectacular strategy was, of course, the first. Never before had insurance companies pushed hospitals and doctors so aggressively for discounts. But the successes would prove Napoleonic—the seeds of defeat were sown on the battlefields of victory. Managed care faced a backlash.

And the Fall

"We were wrong."—*J. D. Kleinke, health-care analyst and best-selling author on the sins of managed care, 2001*

What a difference nine years can make. When Howard Dean lost New Hampshire in 2004, his main Democratic opponent, John Kerry, sounded a populist note: "I'm running for President to free our government from the dominance of the lobbyists, the drug industry, big oil, and HMOs—so that we can give America back its future and its soul."[5] HMOs were now in the same bad company as lobbyists and big oil.

Aetna, as we noted, became the largest health insurance player in America by betting on managed care. By the end of the 1990s, however, it all fell apart. Between shareholder angst and diminished profitability, Aetna was forced to change everything: its CEO, the name of the company, and, yes, the emphasis on HMOs. Today, its enrollment is back down to about thirteen million. The health economist James Robinson summarizes Aetna's trajectory:

> Throughout the turbulent 1990s Aetna was the poster child for the aspirations and failures of managed care, channeling patients and physicians into health maintenance organizations (HMOs); holding down premiums so that enrollment would grow; acquiring competitors to penetrate new markets; and then floundering in adverse publicity, economic shortfalls, and investor disenchantment.[6]

As fast as HMOs had come to dominate American health care, the experiment collapsed. In the 1990s, politicians and business executives had touted HMOs as the savior of American health care. But between 1997 and 2000, HMO enrollment in cities like Miami and Seattle, once hotbeds of managed care, had dropped by as much as 25 percent. And these statistics do not take account of the changes within HMOs themselves. As Debra Draper and colleagues note in *Health Affairs,* the remaining HMOs offer products that look strikingly similar to non-HMO policies.[7] In other words, HMOs stopped functioning like HMOs.

Of course, managed care had not disappeared. By 2004, HMO enrollment, though down 12 percent since the late 1990s, still stood at 70 million. Indemnity plans, once the standard for health insurance, accounted for less than 5 percent of employer-sponsored health insurance. Preferred provider organizations (PPOs) and other types of managed care covered most of working America and their families. But no one was looking to HMOs as the solution to America's health-care troubles. In the American experience with health insurance, never before has an idea so quickly reshaped the landscape only to disappear from it almost overnight.

There are three observations to make about HMOs, in order of increasing controversy:

1. Costs were contained

The basic point of managed care was always to address America's growing health-care bill. Managed care (in particular, HMOs, its most restrictive form) was about managing cost. From this perspective, managed care worked.

In the early 1990s, many people fretted about rising health expenditures. Health care cost about 13.7 percent of the GDP in 1993. The Congressional Budget Office feared the worst—they assumed that costs would continue to rise and that spending would hit 18.9 percent by the end of the decade. Yet by the late 1990s, health spending had increased by slightly less than the overall growth of the economy, leaving expenditures at about 13 percent. That may not seem very significant, but it amounts to $300 billion less than the projection—or, $2,000 in savings for every privately insured patient.

In the private insurance market, where managed care had the greatest pull, premiums remained relatively stable in the mid to late 1990s—in stark contrast to today. During the heyday of managed care, private health spending per capita grew at a modest rate. In 1996, the annual growth was just 2.0 percent; in 2002, after the backlash against managed care, it was 9.6 percent, nearly four times greater than the overall growth in the economy.[8] In terms of hospital costs, the managed-care muscle was obvious: hospital spending actually *dropped* through much of the mid-1990s. In 1997, it fell by an astonishing 5.3 percent.[9]

The Impact of Managed Care:
Annual Change per Capita in Health Care Spending

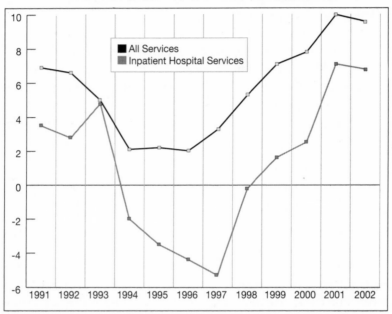

Source: Center for Studying Health System Change

2. Quality of care didn't suffer

Managed care may have held the line on spending, but did patients suffer as a result? Critics had once suggested that American health care was indifferent to cost; now they asserted that it was insensitive to quality. Life under managed care, it seemed, was nasty, brutish, and short. Many in the media found examples to illustrate the point. Perhaps the best-publicized case of HMO denial involved Nelene Fox, a 38-year-old California woman with breast cancer. In 1992, she tried to get coverage for a bone-marrow transplant. Her HMO denied the claim. Fox died a short time afterward—and her grieving family sued, winning a landmark judgment of $89 million.

The Fox case appeared to be just the tip of the iceberg. "Is Your Doctor Looking Out for You? Or Your Insurer?" asked the *Philadelphia Inquirer* (March 24, 1996). "Teacher Battles Cancer and Bureaucracy," noted the *Syracuse Post-Standard* (January 22, 1996). Columnist Bob Herbert of the *New York Times* wrote often on the horrors of HMOs, including an op-ed detailing the story of a man with cancer attempting to get lifesaving treatment, only to be thwarted by his HMO.[10] The backlash made it into the popular culture. In the movie *As Good As It Gets,* a single mother breaks into profanity when her HMO is mentioned. Her sympathetic physician responds: "Actually, I think that's their technical name." Audiences across America burst into applause.

But the literature hardly paints such a damning case. In his book on managed care, *The Economic Evolution of American Health Care,* Prof. David Dranove of Northwestern University reviews the literature and highlights several studies:[11]

- A 1996 study by Fred Hellinger reviewing published literature on HMO quality, finding few measurable differences between managed care and indemnity insurance for a variety of outcome measures.
- A review by Robert Miller and Harold Luft of thirty-five studies published between 1993 and 1997, finding that "Fears that HMOs uniformly lead to worse quality of care are not supported by the evidence.... Hopes that HMOs would improve overall quality also are not supported."
- A 1998 Johns Hopkins University review of cardiovascular care, concluding that "the HMOs studied provided as good, and in some cases better, quality than the non-HMO settings studied."

Even the case of Nelene Fox merits a second look. Yes, she wanted a bone-marrow transplant, and yes, she did succumb to cancer, but many details were glossed over. For one thing, Fox did get the transplant, relying on charitable support to finance it. But bone-marrow transplantation for advanced breast cancer has never been shown to be useful; indeed, a decade later no oncologist would suggest it.

No doubt, some HMOs deserved the bad reputation they earned. On the whole, however, the evidence suggests that widespread stories of HMO cruelty were more Hollywood than reality.

3. It wasn't really so bad

In a Gallup poll asking people to rank the ethical standards of twenty-three different professions, HMO managers ranked second to last, behind journalists and politicians, and only (barely) ahead of car salesmen.[12] When a 1999 Harris poll asked Americans how they felt about different industries, only 34 percent said that managed care did "a good job of servicing the customers" and 37 percent believed that managed care could be trusted "to do the right thing" if they "had a serious safety problem with one of their products or services."[13] In contrast, 47 percent of Americans viewed big oil as trustworthy.

If the judgment is harsh, the exact reason remains less clear. The perception is that HMOs made arbitrary, unappealable decisions about patient care. Researchers at the RAND think tank looked at appeals data from two California HMOs between 1998 and 2000.[14] Most appeals involved the scope of coverage or a member's choice of physician or hospital. Only one-third of the conflicts involved a determination of "medical necessity" and these were concentrated in a handful of medical procedures "that are generally regarded as non-essential."[15] In fact, 57 percent of the disputes over surgeries involved whether or not people would be covered for gastric bypass, breast alteration, or varicose vein removal. Appeals were anything but predetermined—about 40 percent of the time, the HMOs reversed their original decision.

Why HMOs Failed

HMOs sparked a stunning consumer rebellion. In short order, the great savior of American health care faced a public outcry, the threat of litigation from trial lawyers, and state regulations restricting their ability to operate. Dr. Michael DeBakey, a pioneering heart surgeon, suggests the cause of the anger: "We would not allow an unqualified clerk to recommend repairs for our car, so why would we settle for one when it comes to our own health?"[16] But that explanation isn't quite fair. As the health-outcome data show, HMOs were hardly run by unqualified managers making arbitrary, reckless decisions.

Why then the rebellion? The advance of consumerist attitudes among the American public. While consumerism has already changed the way we live, work, and play, the institution of medicine itself has remained remarkably paternalistic. Howard Dean, chairman of the Democratic National Committee, once claimed: "There is no such thing as an informed consumer of health care."[17] But times are changing. Americans aren't heeding the good doctor's advice—increasingly, they treat health care like all other services. They expect to get what they want, when they want it. This attitude, unremarkable in itself, is alien to the dominant health-care paradigm of the last half century.

The Internet helped spark this revolution, empowering people with information and options. The proliferation of Internet pharmacies is one example. The Food and Drug Administration has repeatedly issued warnings about their safety, but Americans aren't listening. With the World Wide Web and FedEx, a Canadian pharmacy offering cheaper prices is just a click away from a patient in Florida or Texas, turning mail-order drugs into a billion-dollar-a-year industry. Or look at the rise of websites devoted to health advice, like WebMD or DrKoop.com. Anyone with computer access can now read the latest abstracts from medical journals on even the most obscure conditions.

Powerful medications like Claritin and Prilosec have already gone over-the-counter. Mevacor, a cholesterol-lowering medication, is also up for review (and has gained approval in Britain). The FDA's comfort with allowing potent drugs to be sold beside cough syrup and vitamins in America's pharmacies reflects the biggest force reshaping health care. MDs no longer have to give scripts; in a way, patients self-prescribe.

In my practice, I've seen firsthand how patient attitudes have evolved in a short time. Patients and their families often enter my office with a thick folder in hand, heavy with clippings and journal abstracts. "We should consider a valproate trial," I will sometimes say to a concerned family. "Yes, we thought you might say that," they will respond, and proceed to quiz me on the latest announcements from the FDA.

As a physician, I remain somewhat ambivalent on the whole trend. Consumerism, after all, isn't always benevolent. For one thing, it lends itself to fads; the rise of "alternative medicine" is a case in point. It's also true that people glean information from both good and bad sources. The Internet is the Wild West of modern medicine—yes, people can find studies from the most prestigious journals and advice from the most august medical bodies, but also offers of snake oil and plenty of misinformation. For better and for worse, American health care is being reshaped by consumerism—and HMOs ran contrary to that trend.

HMO proponents have long argued that their idea was judged unfairly. Alain Enthoven, the Stanford professor and intellectual force behind the rise of HMOs, relates a positive experience of his own. His wife had a hip replacement just a few years back. The HMO worked hard to get her out of hospital quickly—and to make sure that she was fine once she was home. Enthoven describes nurses from the hospital coming to inspect his house and make it "patient friendly."[18] It's difficult not to like the story: everyone involved works to keep costs low, with good health outcomes. "We all buy in," Enthoven notes.[19] But the professor had a choice: his university offered several plans and he picked the HMO. Herein lies the biggest problem with managed care. Americans didn't really have a choice about buying in; their employers enrolled them. The resulting dissatisfaction can be explained by what psychologists call the *lottery effect.*

In the 1960s, a group of researchers conducted a simple experiment. Two groups of people were given lottery tickets and then asked to assess their odds of winning. The first group was simply assigned a ticket. The second group was given a choice—though the tickets were from the same lottery, they could pick one of five. When people from the first group were asked about their chance of winning, they estimated the odds to be infinitesimally low. The second group, asked the exact same question, assumed their odds of winning to be significantly higher. In other words, by choosing their ticket, they felt empowered.

HMOs may have kept up their part of the bargain: quality care at reasonable prices. But Americans rejected the implicit paternalism. That makes sense; in almost every other area of life, Americans are assertive consumers. The managed-care gambit— place control in the hands of bureaucrats—ultimately proved as unpopular as a similar initiative would be concerning some other basic need. Henry Ford told his customers that they could have a car of any color as long as it was black. When he didn't change his business, Americans went elsewhere. Likewise, when HMO bureaucrats told their patients that they could go to any family doctor they wanted as long as it was the one they were assigned, Americans promptly called Human Resources, and then their congressman.

But if Nixon was ultimately wrong—if HMOs would not save American health care—where to look for an alternative?

FOUR

The Third Way

PAM WIMBISH IS AN odd sort of celebrity. She has never penned a novel, founded a charity, or built up a profitable business. She works as a furniture saleswoman in Aurora, Illinois, and contents herself with a relatively quiet family life. But she has been the subject of a press release by a major corporation; House Speaker Dennis Hastert featured her in a press conference; the President of the United States highlighted her in a speech and invited her to the White House for her birthday.

What made her so famous? Ms. Wimbish bought health insurance.

The post-managed-care world is not unlike the Eastern bloc after the Berlin Wall fell: a state of confusion reigns, where people agree on their dislike for the past system but are unsure how to proceed. Many Americans are now enrolled in managed-care-lite insurance plans. In some ways, it's a case of back-to-the-future. Without the discipline of HMOs, double-digit premium increases have returned—and employers drop coverage (increasing the number of uninsured Americans) or hold down wages (increasing the number of unsatisfied Americans). As well, it's difficult to argue that collectively we are significantly healthier despite the higher costs. Some health economists have begun to speak again of "flat-of-the-curve medicine."[1] Managed care collapsed—but is it possible to contain health spending without the paternalism that Americans resent? Consumer-driven health care offers an alternative.

So we find the source of Pam Wimbish's celebrity. She was the first person in America to buy a health savings account, a new type of coverage that could help transform American health care.

Operating in the Dark (and an Alternative)

We know the trouble with the present system—the dearth of competition, leading to high-cost, low-satisfaction medicine. Some advocate putting consumers more in charge of their own health care. Give consumers more control by giving them health dollars to spend, and good things such as innovation will follow. This concept can be loosely called consumer-driven health care—which, like many labels, means different things to different people. Still, the fundamental idea is simple: health care shouldn't be something *done to* Americans. But do consumers have enough information to take control?

Here's an interesting problem: Which hospital would you pick when you need medical help? A Manhattan colleague posed the question to me after a bout of bad health. He awoke one night with pain in his side. Having trained and interned in New York, he was intimately familiar with the different options. He decided to go to Cornell and was diagnosed with appendicitis. By afternoon, he was under the knife.

New York City has its share of hospitals. My colleague could have picked New York Presbyterian, as Bill Clinton did when his heart ailed him. There is Mount Sinai Medical Center, the pioneering institution whose staff have discovered and described more than a dozen different diseases. But he picked Cornell. Why? "It has a good reputation, I think."

What's remarkable is that my friend is so much more connected and informed than a typical New York patient, yet his choice of Cornell's ER was based on practically no information. He didn't look at outcomes or cost analyses. He essentially picked a hospital on a whim. But then, what else could he have done? Just because he's a doctor doesn't mean he has much more information about hospitals than the rest of us.

Contrast his largely blind decision with something less dramatic—a choice of hotels in Manhattan. Again, there is a rich array of options, from the opulent Waldorf Astoria to the utilitarian Holiday Inn. Business travelers and tourists have much information about these options at their fingertips. Visit sites like hotels.com, and you find photos, star ratings, and value-for-money recommendations in abundance. For those who are technologically challenged, the local bookstore offers a sea of information with its Fodor guides and the like. As Prof. Regina Herzlinger of Harvard observes, "the market is driven to give information."[2] How different this is from health care! For a relatively unimportant decision, there is a wealth of information, but for a major health decision, even doctors are in the dark.

Granted, in the case of my colleague with sharp abdominal pain, it would have been difficult to cost out different options and carefully weigh the choices. But in an ideal world, people would be armed with information, like basic surgery outcomes and mortality rates. A patient in need of, say, a hip replacement would then look at his options and make a choice, not unlike a tourist selecting a hotel. In fact, Aetna now offers a website with information on hospitals for its participants.

To Regina Herzlinger, this makes sense; she argues that consumer-driven health care is the future. But the Harvard professor is a bit of an iconoclast. In the heyday of managed care, she established herself as a skeptic. In 1989, she penned an essay for the *Harvard Business Review* predicting the collapse of managed care; two years later, she advanced a similar argument in the *Atlantic Monthly*—whose editors, incidentally, were so uncomfortable with her point that they tried to soften the tone.

Time proved Herzlinger right. "Managed care is out," she says.[3] People—and particularly the people making decisions about health benefits for companies—are looking for an alternative. Some companies are lobbying for a Canadian-style system. But Herzlinger believes that a more realistic option, one that is in synch with American values, is consumer-directed health care.

Imagine a patient with grade 2 congestive heart failure, she suggests. He should be able to choose a clinic that specializes in exactly this—with data available on health outcomes and cost. Beyond this, Herzlinger sees people having control over their benefits (like wanting long-term care), the extent of their coverage (say, $5 million rather than $1 million in total coverage), the length of the insurance term (say, five years rather than just one), and the providers involved.

In other words, Prof. Herzlinger envisions a radically different health-care system. And we have already taken the first step to get there.

A Step in the Right Direction

"I not only believe consumer-driven health plans are the best solution to our health care crisis, it's probably the only sustainable solution that's not going to lead to a single-payer system."— *John Mackey, CEO of Whole Foods*[4]

As outlined in the last chapter, the most basic problem with U.S. health care is that Americans don't really pay for the care they receive. How to address this? The beginning of wisdom can be found in the Nixon administration.

We saw how Nixon White House policy enabled the rise of HMOs; ironically, the most promising alternative to managed care also comes from that administration. In 1974, Jesse Hixson and Paul Worthington, two economists with the Social Security Administration, developed the idea of "health banks." With traditional (indemnity) insurance and HMOs, Americans were overinsured and thus insulated from the consequences of their health-care decisions. Hixson and Worthington proposed an alternative: Employers would deposit money for health care directly into the savings accounts of employees at specially chartered health banks. For smaller expenses, employees could draw on their accounts; for catastrophic events, the bank would pool multiple deposits and thus be able to offer loans if an employee's account was insufficient to cover the medical bills.

Hixson went on to work for the American Medical Association, eventually becoming its principal economist. He continued to promote the idea of involving employees more in health decisions. He found a supporter in John Goodman at the National Center for Policy Analysis in Dallas. Goodman was initially excited by the prospect of using individual accounts—modified IRAs—to reform Medicare. He developed the idea further and in 1990 organized a task force with representatives from academia, think tanks, and business. Drawing on the task force's report, Goodman wrote *Patient Power* with the economist Gerald Musgrave in 1992.

A detailed book of nearly seven hundred pages, full of technical jargon and a plethora of statistics, *Patient Power* hardly seems like a bestseller type of book—and yet it was, selling over 300,000 copies. It comments on various topics, including Canadian health care, the need for rural medical enterprise zones, and challenges for the individual health insurance market, to name a few. But the main idea for employer-sponsored insurance is simple: Employees would get tax-free dollars to pay for their smaller health-care expenses and would have a high-deductible insurance for catastrophic events. This would leave the bulk of spending decisions to individuals.

A businessman named Pat Rooney heard Gerald Musgrave give a lecture and became a convert. Rooney offered medical savings accounts (MSAs) to his employees at Golden Rule Insurance. Impressed by the popularity of this type of health insurance, he began marketing it to other companies. Rooney and Goodman worked tirelessly to promote the MSA concept.

While MSAs were gaining purchase in the imagination of America's polity, the business world remained unconvinced. Golden Rule Insurance sold plans to small employers, while a few big companies, like Quaker Oats and Forbes, offered MSA plans to their employees. But these efforts were limited by tax law. Unlike employer-paid premiums, MSA deposits were subject to income and payroll taxes, and unspent funds could not be rolled over. Fortunately, interest in MSAs was robust on Capitol Hill. Congressman Bill Archer, a Republican and chairman of the House Ways and Means Committee, championed the idea and favored a tax-code change. Working with his Democratic colleague Andy Jacobs, Archer amended the Kennedy-Kassebaum bill (Health Insurance Portability and Accountability Act) of 1996 to include a provision making MSAs tax-free for the self-employed and small businesses. MSAs were a Washington answer to the mess of American health care. They offered a clear alternative to the paternalism of managed care—people would be empowered with health dollars. Conservatives enthused that MSAs would change every-thing; liberals fretted that MSAs might just do so. But for all the debate and discussion, it would be difficult to think of another health reform initiative that affected so few. MSAs were doomed from the beginning.

"The legislation was just too limiting," explains John Good-man, president of the National Center for Policy Analysis and an MSA advocate.[5] It restricted MSAs to small businesses (those with fewer than fifty employees) and individuals, and was overly rigid as to the way MSAs must be structured. Making the situa-tion worse, MSAs were approved as an "experiment," lasting just four years. Congress capped enrollment at 750,000 people; fewer than 100,000 signed up. Congress extended the experiment, but MSAs were a flop. In 2003, Congress made a second effort. As a last-minute addition to the Medicare Modernization Act, aimed at gaining the support of congressional conservatives, House Ways and Means chairman Bill Thomas added provisions creat-ing Health Savings Accounts (HSAs). These are freer in structure than MSAs and, more importantly, they are permanent. "HSAs," notes Greg Scandlen of Consumers for Health Care Choice, "are the little idea that could transform health care."[6]

Anyone—mom-and-pop operations, large corporations, indi-viduals—can open a health savings account. HSAs allow people to purchase a relatively inexpensive high-deductible insurance and deposit money into a tax-free account. HSAs, thus, marry real insurance (that is, coverage for high and unpredictable costs) with contributions to a savings account that can be used to pay for smaller health expenses and "rolled over" from year to year. For companies and individuals looking to avoid high-cost health insurance, HSAs are immediately attractive. After all, low-deductible insurance is expensive and any move away from this concept (really, prepaid health care rather than health insurance) is going to reduce premiums. The economist Martin Feldstein noted in the *Wall Street Journal* that a typical Blue Cross of Cali-fornia family policy cost $8,460, with a $500 deductible per mem-ber.[7] But a similar HSA policy costs just $3,936, with a $2,500 deductible—so the difference in savings ($4,524) actually exceeds the maximum additional out-of-pocket expense that the family would face if they reached the maximum deductible. The HSA approach results in great savings. Data from eHealthInsurance, a leading online insurance brokerage, suggest that a majority (55 percent) of customers purchasing health insurance through the HSA approach pay less than a hundred dollars a month.[8]

HSA 101

What is an HSA?
Every HSA has two components:
  1. A personal savings account
  2. A catastrophic health insurance policy with a high deductible

How high is a high deductible?
For 2006, catastrophic coverage with a high deductible is defined by law as at least $1,050 for individuals and $2,100 for families.

How much can be deposited in the tax-free account?
The purchaser can deposit up to $2,700 for individuals or $5,450 for families per year, or the value of their deductible, whichever is less. Note: the law also allows people age 55–65 to top up their contributions by $500 per year, indexed to inflation.

For individuals, HSAs help level the tax-code playing field. Remember, employers can pay for health insurance in pretax dollars, but individuals cannot. With an HSA, the contribution to the medical account is in pretax dollars. "This was a no-brainer," Wimbish said of her insurance policy purchase. "One hundred percent of the deductible can go to the HSA for any medical expense, even ones that may not be covered by the policy. It's funded with pre-tax dollars, and as a self-employed person, I'm always looking for ways to save money."[9]

The bigger hope for HSAs, though, is that they will create a market for health services. With Americans thinking of health care in consumerist terms, HSAs sound ideal: move decisions to individuals at a time when, increasingly, they demand just that. At present, third-party payment means—as Nelson Sabatini observes—that Americans are buying health services with someone else's credit card. John Cogan, a Hoover Institution fellow, summarizes the situation before HSAs: "Consumers have little incentive to limit their use of unnecessary medical care, little incentive to shop for the health plan that best suits their needs, and little incentive to evaluate their care on the basis of value."[10]

Pam Wimbish illustrates how HSAs may address this problem. According to an article in the *Wall Street Journal,* she developed foot pain a month after signing on to the plan.[11] It turned out that a screw in her foot from a previous surgery had come loose. Like any savvy consumer, Ms. Wimbish took charge of the situation and thought about what she really needed. When a simple day-surgery procedure was suggested, she looked around and decided on a local surgery center. She asked about clinic fees and offered to pay upfront—thereby getting a 50 percent discount. When she found out that an anesthetist would come in specifically to do the foot block, she asked her surgeon just to do it. She also negotiated the surgeon's compensation down from $1,260 to $630. Finally, she got a prescription from her doctor for both antibiotics and painkillers, but only filled the former. "In the past, my attitude would have been, 'Just have all the prescriptions filled because insurance was paying for it, whether or not I need them.'"[12]

As employers increasingly fret over rising health costs, consumer-driven plans offer a way to hold the line on spending without forcing employees into managed care. Many employers haven't signed on to the idea. One who has is John Mackey, the founder and CEO of Whole Foods, which has 162 stores in three countries and is considered the fastest-growing grocery chain in America. Mr. Mackey first heard of this type of health insurance in the most unlikely of places: on the Appalachian Trail. He was taking a five-month sabbatical hiking the Appalachians when, on one of his occasional stops to catch up on e-mail and news, he read about an IRS ruling that allowed health reimbursement accounts (HRAs), a forerunner to HSAs.[13]

If consumer-driven health care seemed like a novel idea to him, it was just what was needed—the Whole Foods self-insured plan was insolvent. Indeed, health costs hit the bottom line. In 2002, earnings were down 5 cents a share. Rather than cut back on benefits, Mackey came up with a new tack: a consumer-driven plan based on HRAs.

When employees complained, Mackey revised his approach. He visited nearly every store to meet with employees and explain the new program, and he made some changes as a result. Ulti-mately, he decided it was his employees' plan so they should be involved in the decision. Employees could vote on all benefits, including a choice of three health plans (two traditional plans and a consumer-driven plan):

> So we had, which is probably unprecedented in corporate Amer-ica, a company-wide vote on our benefits in summer 2003. We let our team members suggest benefits they'd like to see, and, my God, you wouldn't believe what they came up with. One suggestion was pet bereavement assistance.... We fixed the number of dollars—we said, "This is how much we're going to pay." Then we costed out each benefit and we let the team mem-bers select the benefits by basically ranking them. The benefits that got the most votes were the ones that we selected for the next three years....
>
> Interestingly enough, when the new health insurance plan was put to the vote, it got an 83% favorable vote.[14]

Key Features of the Whole Foods Plan

No premiums
After a few months on the job, individual workers get free coverage. For the families of workers, free coverage starts after about five years.

High deductibles
$500 for prescriptions and $1,000 for all other medical costs.

Employee accounts
Whole Foods deposits $300 to $1,800 per year, depending on length of employment, to help meet the deductible.

Results
Overall medical claims fell 13 percent in the first year. About 90 percent of employees had money left over to use next year. Claims rose in the second year—but overall health costs have risen just 3 percent per annum and total costs per employee are well below most company plans.

Source: John Mackey, *Wall Street Journal.*

Whole Foods' health costs have gone up only about 3 per-cent annually since the introduction of a consumer-driven plan, as opposed to the double-digit increases experienced by most other companies. Just as importantly, the plan is popular. Because many employees don't have to pay an explicit premium with the new insurance, about 95 percent of eligible workers are enrolled, up from about 65 percent who participated in Whole Foods' health insurance programs in 2002.[15]

HSAs could create a market for health services, thereby reducing costs and increasing innovation. Although Prof. Herzlinger's vision of a competitive market for health services is a long way off, health savings accounts are a first step there. And they are enjoying some early successes:

- In January 2006, America's Health Insurance Plans, a trade group, released a survey of its membership showing that enrollment in HSAs had tripled over the previous six months and exceeded three million Americans. About half are in the individual insurance market.
- A Blue Cross survey found high levels of satisfaction among HSA holders: 65 percent would recommend the plan to a friend.
- More and more insurance companies offer the plans. Blue-Cross BlueShield promises HSA products in forty-nine states this year. Even Kaiser Permanente, the company that invented managed care, now markets HSAs.
- Large employers are increasingly looking at the option. A Mercer study found that 5 percent of employers with over 500 employees and 22 percent of companies with over 20,000 employees were offering these consumer-driven plans in 2005. Next year, 11 percent of all employers will offer such plans, including Wal-Mart.

Responding to the Critics

The idea of health savings accounts—and the consumer-driven health care that they represent—has elicited howls of opposition from some quarters. Here are the three strongest criticisms, and responses to them.

Criticism 1: People are too ignorant to make their own health decisions.

In a *New York Times* essay, Hillary Clinton suggested that "instead of putting consumers in the driver's seat," the health savings

Five Companies That Are Transforming American Health Care
(and that you've never heard of)

DEFINITY HEALTH

Definity Health has just a dozen clients. But don't let that deceive you—they include Fortune 500 companies like Medtronic, Siemens, and Amazon.com. Definity Health helps these corporate clients manage their health benefits by building consumer-driven options. To assist subscribers, Definity Health provides consumers with medical pricing information, a consumer medical library, hospital quality ratings, and a health-coaching program. It's a potent cocktail, and Definity Health has an impressive record, holding health spending growth to 3 percent a year. Others have taken note—and in November 2004, UnitedHealth bought the company. Definity Health will continue to run under its own name.

DESTINY HEALTH

Destiny Health is based on a successful business model—its parent company in South Africa markets the most popular medical savings account plan. Destiny Health offers more than a standard HSA/HRA. In order to promote wellness, the company has a point-based system to encourage intelligent choices—like getting routine physical exams and other types of preventive care, or joining a gym. Members who accrue enough points can cash out for rewards.

VIVIUS

Some insurance companies simply assign you a group of doctors. Vivius offers an alternative: it allows employees to design their own provider networks, choosing family doctors, specialists, and even hospitals, and setting the copayment rate. Thus, an asthmatic would be able to pick a specific respirologist. The interactive website then costs out the health premium, calculating the payroll deduction.

THE LEAPFROG GROUP

There can't be much consumerism unless patients are armed with good information. My colleague, for instance, made an arbitrary choice when he needed hospital care. The Leapfrog Group is hoping to take the guesswork out of this type of decision. Collecting data on high-risk surgeries, the Leapfrog Group makes comparisons (and, perhaps one day, comparison shopping) possible.

eHEALTHINSURANCE

Not that long ago, insurance companies thought little of the individual insurance market. But as more and more Americans find themselves without employer-funded health coverage, hundreds of thousands of people are interested in buying a policy for themselves and their families. But how to pick a plan? Enter eHealthInsurance. "We find the right health insurance to meet people's needs," explains CEO Gary Lauer. The company offers an easy-to-use website that allows anyone to enter his or her Zip Code, list out some demographic information, and then get dozens of insurance options, with pricing and details. Over 150 insurance companies are participating. For those with Internet-phobia, there's also a 1-800 number.

account "actually leaves consumers at the mercy of a broken market. This system shifts the costs, the risks and the burdens of disease onto the individuals who have the misfortune of being sick." The senator went on to ask: "Think about the times you have been sick or injured—were you able under those circumstances to negotiate for the best price or shop for the best care?"[16] Along similar lines, Congressman Pete Stark of California argued that patients either "feel they are invincible" if healthy, or else, when sick, are "absolutely brain dead, sniveling, begging and fantasizing ills and pains."[17]

This argument has merit, but it is contradicted by data. The RAND think tank in California tracked two thousand families over eight years in a study that cost about a quarter of a billion dollars (adjusting for inflation)—one of the most expensive experiments in the history of social science. The study compared the health and the health-care spending of two groups: one with free health care, the other with some type of cost sharing up to a certain point, after which a catastrophic insurance kicked in (structurally not unlike an HSA). The result? Those on the free plan cost 40 percent more but in the end were no healthier than those on the HSA-style plan. This suggests that people are able to make intelligent health-care choices when provided with a financial incentive to do so. Indeed, the parallel between the RAND experiment and the design of consumer-driven health-care plans is not lost on the study's prime mover, Prof. Joseph Newhouse.[18]

Returning to Senator Clinton's point, people obviously aren't going to call around for a good price on care after being involved in a major car accident. But most of medicine is not emergency care. People could intelligently respond to better incentives in most situations.

Of course, there are limits to just how savvy an individual patient may be. Critics suggest that even if people can make good choices in easy cases—like deciding not to go to the hospital with a common cold, but opting for the local ER with serious chest pain—they can't make rational decisions in most medical situations. How would a nonclinician find the best value when choosing a cholesterol medication? How would he or she interpret test results?

Already, though, the market has begun to respond to the information asymmetry. Many insurance companies aren't just selling the health savings accounts; they're offering companion services, like information websites. At the Cigna site, for example, members can estimate annual costs, compare drug prices, and get comparisons of hospitals (showing quality ratings for certain procedures as well as the cost and length of stay). Other companies offer "health coaches," so that a health professional can guide patients along, helping them navigate the choppy waters of health care. Companies outside the insurance industry are also getting involved. Websites such as DestinationRx.com and PharmacyChecker.com let patients search for their medication and compare prices at different online pharmacies.

Criticism 2: HSAs help the wealthy shelter their money.

In testimony before the Joint Economic Committee in Congress, Gail Shearer argued:

> Expansion of medical savings accounts (MSAs) under the new name of Health Savings Accounts (HSAs) adds a new wrinkle to "consumer-driven health care" plans by making the contributions to the health reimbursement account tax deductible. This new tax policy, combined with high deductible health coverage, is likely to appeal disproportionately to the healthy and wealthy.
> - The healthy benefit because they have the new prospect of a tax-sheltered investment in which money is not taxed when put in or when withdrawn.
> - The wealthy, with higher tax brackets, benefit disproportionately because the tax savings are larger at higher tax brackets than at lower tax brackets.[19]

This criticism is cited often, suggesting that HSAs are nothing more than a tax giveaway or, to use slightly more technical language, that they amount to regressive taxation.

What opponents of HSAs fail to mention, though, is that the tax code is already quite biased. Tax fairness is built on the principle of horizontal equity—that is, people who have the same ability to pay tax should pay the same amount of tax. Clearly, the present tax code violates this principle in spades. As assistant director of the Congressional Budget Office, Rosemary Marcuss listed the ways in testimony before the Senate Finance Committee:

> People with employment-based health insurance pay less tax than do otherwise similar people without insurance. Self-employed people and those who are out of the work force receive no benefit from the tax exclusion. People whose employers provide more expensive health insurance coverage receive a greater benefit than people with less generous coverage. People whose employers pay a larger share of their health insurance premiums receive a greater benefit than people whose employers pay a smaller share.[20]

As noted in Chapter Two, the tax exclusion also violates the principle of vertical equity—that is, people with more ability to pay tax should pay more tax. A family earning between $20,000 and $30,000 gets just a $725 tax break; in contrast, those with incomes above $100,000 get $2,780.

Health savings accounts hardly make the situation worse. In fact, as Ms. Wimbish has noted, they allow those who don't get coverage from their employers to gain a tax break. HSAs thus provide a bit of horizontal equity. Also, since contributions to the health accounts are capped, they are slightly less biased toward higher income levels than the pre-HSA tax code.

Criticism 3: HSAs punish the chronically ill and the uninsured.

Economist David Cutler summarizes this argument: "Some see HSAs as vehicles for rich and healthy people to be in different plans [and insurance pools] than poorer, sicker people."[21] The claim that HSAs will "drain the insurance pool" builds on exaggerated fears that HSAs will attract only wealthy and healthy individuals, leaving the sick and the poor behind in what's left of the insurance market, and thereby forcing more and more expensive premiums on those least able to pay.

The flaw in this "adverse selection" argument is that there really is no such nationwide pool of insured people that cross-subsidizes each other's premiums.[22] Actually, employers—usually large ones—tend to self-insure. That is, they constitute their own separate insurance pool of employees and their families. Premiums are based on what the group actually spends on health care. For those who are not self-insured—that is, for most small and medium-sized employers—insurance premiums are based on recent medical claims cost experiences, or "experience rating." In fact, insurance pooling is even more fragmented. Insurance companies do not cross-subsidize each other. Even within large insurance carriers there are separate pools across different states and for various types of customers.

Health savings accounts, thus, wouldn't shatter the fragile communal insurance pool, but merely provide options for people. For the uninsured, in particular, health savings accounts are probably quite attractive given their lower cost. According to the online insurance brokerage eHealthInsurance, nearly half of their HSA customers earn less than $50,000 a year. A full 70 percent pay under $100 a month for the coverage. One-third were previously uninsured.[23] Assurant Health, a large insurer, notes that many new HSA purchasers are over forty, often with chronic health problems.

Building a Market for Health Care

Like all aspects of the human experience, health care is colored by trends. For a time, government expansion was the buzz. (Recall that the American Medical Association and no fewer than twenty-three Republican senators actually signed on to Hillary Clinton's vision of employer-mandated coverage.) Then the excitement was all for managed care. Today, some of the same people who once waxed poetic about HMOs now enthuse about HSAs. "Transformational" and "revolutionary" are words often heard. Writing in *Health Affairs,* the economist Tom Miller summarizes the situation wittily:

> "Consumer-driven" vehicles remain the hot new items in this year's showroom for health care reform. Whether they are built on the chassis of a new health savings account (HSA), powered by a late-model health reimbursement arrangement (HRA), or offered in a multiple-choice menu of insurance plans using hybrid fuels, consumer-drive health plans are drawing the most

attention, if not the most sales. Even older product lines of health insurance and health treatments are being repackaged under labels such as "consumer driven," "consumer directed," or "consumer choice."[24]

A bit of perspective is needed. The beginning and end of health reform didn't occur when President Bush signed the Medicare bill of 2003 into law. HSAs will not single-handedly change the way Americans access health care, but they are part of an opening wedge, altering how employers, employees, and providers view health care. Likewise, while the larger concept of consumer-driven health care is important, it is not the end of the road for health reform, but rather, perhaps, the end of the beginning.

To push America more on the path to a market for health care, major changes are needed. The creation of HSAs was a good start, but much work remains to be done. Like a Latin American country that has just voted out its socialist government, there is opportunity for significant change. There is also potential to discredit the whole movement and end up pushing Americans even further down the path to a government-managed health-care system.

Here are some important steps that must be taken:

Step 1: Make HSAs popular.

Though created by law in 2003, health savings accounts are still novel, and a relatively small slice of the health insurance marketplace. Tom Miller observes:

> Many potential buyers are still mostly kicking the tires and waiting to see how test drives by others on the lot turn out. Most of them traded in their drab HMOs several years ago, because they were hard to squeeze into, wouldn't take them where they wanted to go, and turned out to be more Hyundai than Honda. But when they moved up to roomier PPO health utility vehicles, keeping those cash guzzlers on the open road sent prices so high that even "a man making a good salary" wondered if he could continue to own one.[25]

While employees and the self-employed haven't exactly rushed out to sign on to the plan, many employers have not added HSAs to their menu of insurance choices. This cool reception is more than disappointing—it's potentially ruinous to the success of HSAs. To create a market for health services, many people need to have HSAs. The neighborhood family physician isn't going to post his fee schedule if only one or two patients in his practice have an HSA. It would be different, though, if one-third of his patients had such coverage.

Here politicians can play a leading role. First and foremost, they can speak about health savings accounts. President Bush has done an excellent job, not simply by promoting HSAs but by signing up for the plan himself.[26] Unfortunately, other national and state leaders have been quiet on the subject. A gubernatorial boost in states like California and New York could double or triple the national enrollment.[27]

There's another potential leadership role: state governments could provide the option to their own employees. Governor Schwarzenegger, for instance, could offer the plan to California's more than a quarter of a million state employees. State agencies, like the University of California, should also be encouraged to offer an HSA option as part of their menu of health plans.

Step 2: Free HSAs.

Drafted at the last minute, the legislation creating HSAs is rigid—the sort of compromise that makes sense to a tax committee of Congress, but not necessarily ideal for the real world. Recognizing this, President Bush in his State of the Union address suggested some small steps to improve HSAs, including the idea of raising the annual contribution amount (at present, a person or his employer can add no more to his health account than the annual deductible of his catastrophic policy).

There is, however, a more fundamental flaw that must be remedied. The HSA structure is too restrictive: the law demands high-deductible insurance for all employees under all circumstances. As John Goodman points out, there are good reasons to treat different circumstances differently—for instance, it may make more sense that a diabetic not face any deductible for hospital care. Goodman suggests that chronic illness itself may benefit from a different tack altogether, with limited deductibles for many services.

Even better than loosening restrictions to allow flexibility in deductibles within plans and among subscribers, why not get the government out of the business of micromanaging health insurance altogether? Allow individuals and companies to allocate a certain amount, pretax, to be used for premiums or health accounts, or both. Insurance companies will then design products with different mixes of health accounts and insurance.

Step 3: Address the regulatory excess.

Architecturally, the cement-and-glass visage of the Arizona Heart Institute is stunning. But what's really amazing is the care that goes on inside. Focused on cardiology and cardiac surgery, this hospital and others in the private MedCath chain of heart hospitals attract more complex cases, treat patients with shorter stays, and yet achieve better outcomes. All this, and the care costs less than at community hospitals. The specialization, in other words, pays off—MedCath has drawn national and international attention. It represents a significant break from the traditional hospital, which attempts to offer everything for everybody. In an age of consumerism, the Arizona Heart Institute would seem to be a model.

Except that Congress doesn't see it that way. The Medicare Modernization Act of 2003 includes an eighteen-month moratorium on reimbursement to new specialty hospitals. Since then, Congress has pushed the moratorium for another three years. As a joint Federal Trade Commission / Department of Justice report suggests, state laws also undermine the establishment of such specialty hospitals.[28] Thus, even if Congress doesn't extend the moratorium, it seems unlikely that the facilities will ever be established in more than seven or eight states. The war against specialty hospitals indicates that politicians, despite the enthusiastic rhetoric about choice in health care—particularly among Republicans—are doing little to tackle the regulations that undermine it. Action would be needed, after all, since government has spent five decades undermining choice and competition in health care.

Americans view health care as a sector of the economy that is largely untouched by government. In fact, the opposite is true—health care is riddled with laws and regulations that govern financing, billing, and basic practice. "The U.S. health care system, while among the most 'market oriented' in the industrialized world, remains the most intensively regulated sector of the U.S. economy," observes Charles Phelps, an economist at the University of Rochester.[29] But here's the problem with the surfeit of rules: HSAs will never flourish as long as the heavy hand of government weighs down on the sector.

Consider some of the federal legislation: STARK, EMTALA, Medicaid, Medicare, FDA regulations, licensing requirements, the Bush I laboratory bill, EPSDT, ERISA. For American hospitals and clinics, Medicare alone requires more than 100,000 pages of regulations to be complied with. Add state legislation to the mix — malpractice law, insurance law and regulations, public-health reporting requirements, drug education, certification of need—and Prof. Phelps' point is easily appreciated. All these requirements have consequences, in terms of both cost and innovation.

Take the Emergency Medical Treatment and Active Labor Act (EMTALA) of 1986, which requires hospitals to treat any patient in an emergency situation, regardless of ability to pay. Singling out this legislation seems absurd, like attacking motherhood and apple pie. But court and government interpretations of the law have resulted in unintended consequences. Because of EMTALA, people happily use ERs for primary care and not just emergencies. Even the definition of entering a hospital has been expanded. Patients in parking lots are now considered to be in the hospital, as are people on driveways and sidewalks. The end result: a bonanza for trial lawyers—and the closure of numerous ERs (sixty in California alone since 1990).[30]

EMTALA is just the tip of the iceberg. The consequences of over-regulation are easy to see. Medicare rules aimed at fairness end up creating a bizarre world of hospital and drug pricing; ownership laws allow hospital monopolies to flourish. These regulations carry a price tag. Using several techniques, Christopher Conover of Duke University estimates the cost of health service regulations at nearly $340 billion a year.[31] Prof. Conover acknowledges that certain rules have beneficial effects, but still estimates that the net cost of health regulations is about $1,500 per year for each household.

Washington, D.C., and the states need to act to address the regulatory excess. Some have suggested another approach. In *Healthy, Wealthy, and Wise: Five Steps to a Better Health Care System,* authors Glenn Hubbard, John Cogan, and Daniel Kessler suggest that the federal government use antitrust laws (and thus lawsuits) to encourage competition.[32] Their approach is not unreasonable—but, to date, practically nothing has come of the much-touted actions against big hospitals. The best way to break monopolistic behavior, it would seem, is through competition.

A FOUR-DAY STRIKE ISN'T exactly the stuff of legends, but the tension between SBC Communication, Inc., and Communications Workers of America (CWA) in the 2004 contract talks says much about health care today. Health benefits were a major point in the negotiations. After double-digit increases in premiums, management proposed a new deal, doubling the copayments for the average employee. The union balked.

Perspective is important: prior to the contract negotiations, the average CWA worker, with annual salaries topping $60,000 a year, didn't pay any direct monthly premium. The proposed copays, incidentally, averaged $70 a month for the employees, as opposed to $35.[33] But in a fight over $35 a month, much is wrong with both sides. For management, the boldest idea to address spiraling health costs was to double the copay. For labor, the response was a knee-jerk rejection.

If American health care is to be substantively changed, there must be a cultural change. People need to rethink the health care they want and their role in obtaining it.

For those receiving coverage from their employers—a majority of Americans—health insurance has been taken for granted. Instilling competition into American health care is a necessary prescription for an ailing patient. But changes aren't needed only from Washington. People need to start asking hard questions when they see their doctor. Employers need to contemplate their role not just as a health payer but as a health manager.

Health savings accounts represent an exciting first step. An executive at Whole Foods tells a great story.[34] He visits his podiatrist because of a longstanding foot problem. The podiatrist starts by suggesting that he walk up and down the hallway so that the specialist can check his gait. When the executive gets the bill, the itemized price for the observation is $50. The executive calls the podiatrist, who drops the charge—and mentions that no patient has ever questioned the fee before. With just a small cost incentive, this individual became a health consumer.

But so much remains to be done. Earlier in this chapter, we outlined Prof. Regina Herzlinger's vision for health care where people have greater ability to customize their benefits—and live with the consequences. It's difficult to see this happening without a significant cultural change. As long as employees and their unions oppose even modest changes, as long as employers can offer little more than cosmetic updates to managed-care-lite plans, her concept of a truly consumer-driven health-care system is as incredible as Jules Verne's novels must have been to his nineteenth-century readers.

Everyone involved must change, not just employers and employees. Insurance companies presently market plans without any attempt at simplifying or standardizing their language, making the comparison of health plans all but impossible.[35] Providers are stuck in a cookie-cutter mold, offering care based on the billing codes developed by the American Medical Association and Medicare's administrators.[36] While medicine has evolved since 1941, health care in many ways has not.

For decades, because of financing arrangements, American health care has been shielded from market forces. The result has been unsatisfactory for all involved. But can the consumerism that works for private insurance apply also to other health-care problems? Would it insure the uninsured, improve Medicare and Medicaid, and give us cheaper and better prescription drugs? In the following chapters, we take the golden key of choice and competition, and use it to unlock these problems.

FIVE

Insuring America

THEY WALK AMONG US: 46 million who lack health insurance. This is a stain on the soul of America. As a doctor, I've seen the angst on their faces; as a person, I've felt the guilt. We know that these citizens are the poorest among us, deprived of basic health care and doomed to struggle with illness and even death that could be prevented. As one advocacy group recently declared: "For millions of low-income Americans, the health care safety net is a myth."[1]

Such is the conventional thinking on the uninsured—the moving prose that works itself into campaign speeches, newspaper columns, and even movies. To better experience the plight of the uninsured, I visited one of the poorest neighborhoods in America—and found a hospital.

Los Angeles County Hospital is hardly an architectural marvel; the building itself is a throwback to the 1920s. The ER is small and awkward. On some wards, patients are packed six to a room, with only dirty curtains separating them from one another. But as one cardiologist told me, "Even if [the hospital] looks like it should be demolished, the acute care is very good."[2] That's an important point: the hospital boasts state-of-the-art care, with a CAT scan and access to an MRI; *U.S. News & World Report* routinely cites a variety of L.A. County departments for providing the best care in America.[3] L.A. County—like hundreds of other hospitals and clinics across the country—is an oasis of charity care.

Yes, there are uninsured Americans; but as my visit to Los Angeles County Hospital illustrated, the problem is very different from what is generally believed. The numbers of uninsured are not so large; their problems, not so dire; and the necessary remedy, not so socialist. A full 93 percent of Americans either are insured or could afford insurance. How to help those without coverage? The single best prescription is to free up the health insurance market, making insurance more affordable, and to focus government spending on those most in need. That may not sound particularly ambitious compared with some other ideas being floated, but it will insure millions more Americans, including the poorest among them.

What We All Know: 46 and 18

There is just one day a year for us to contemplate the achievements of George Washington and Abraham Lincoln, but Americans have a full week to weigh the issue of the uninsured, thanks to the generous funding of the Robert Wood Johnson Foundation. Since 2003, organizations across the country participate in Cover the Uninsured Week, chaired by former presidents Carter and Ford. The participants are diverse, including the American Medical Association, Families USA, and the Mennonite Church. If some of the 1,200 or so activities planned during the week seem odd (the candlelight vigils and interfaith prayers, for instance), this much is clear: regardless of ideological stripe or vested self-interest, everyone worries about the uninsured.

Cover the Uninsured Week may be more carnival and PR than public policy. But if one issue unsettles Americans about their health-care system, the lack of universal coverage is it. No discussion of health insurance is complete without some mention of those who don't have it. PBS documentaries lament the "crisis" of the uninsured; magazines profile their hard-luck stories; politicians claim their plight as the impetus for change and a host of prescriptions.

Senator Hillary Clinton, for example, cited just one statistic in her sprawling *New York Times* essay to illustrate the deficiencies of American health care—the number of uninsured Americans:

> In 1993, there were 37 million uninsured Americans. In the late
> 90's, the situation improved slightly, largely because of the
> improved economy and the passage of the Children's Health
> Insurance Program. But now some 4[6] million Americans are
> uninsured . . . .[4]

For Senator Clinton—and for many others—the number of
uninsured is a barometer for measuring the failings of the system. Even a calm, sensible centrist like Matthew Miller, a former
Clinton adviser and a senior fellow at the Center for American
Progress, grows edgy when discussing the uninsured:

> The uninsured may seem invisible, but today their ranks are
> equal to the combined populations of Oklahoma, Connecticut,
> Iowa, Mississippi, Kansas, Arkansas, Utah, Nevada, New Mexico,
> West Virginia, Nebraska, Idaho, Maine, New Hampshire, Hawaii,
> Rhode Island, Montana, Delaware, North Dakota, South Dakota,
> Alaska, Vermont and Wyoming. Would America conceivably turn
> its back on the citizens of twenty-three states if they lacked
> basic health coverage? That is what we've been doing for
> decades.[5]

The strong rhetoric focuses on one central point: it's wrong
for anyone to be without health insurance. Two numbers often
appear to back up this point: 46 and 18. The commonly quoted
number of uninsured is 46 million; among those without coverage, 18,000 apparently die every year because of poor health care.
    The issue of the uninsured, however, is much more com-
plex. Indeed, much of what people assume—including the 46 million and 18,000 figures—turns out to be misleading. Here are five
major myths about the uninsured.

Myth 1: The number of uninsured is spiraling up.

"Record Level of Americans Not Insured on Health," blared a *New
York Times* headline in 2004.[6] Almost no discussion of the uninsured
is complete without mentioning the "growing" scale of the problem. Newspapers like the *Times* not only quote the numbers but
often include scary-looking graphs demonstrating that the number
of uninsured has been rising year after year, now hitting 46 million.

But there are two ways to look at this numbers: first, as a raw number (simply the number of people who lack insurance); second, as a percentage of the population as a whole. The problem-is-growing experts quote the raw numbers and ignore the percentages.

It is true that the number of uninsured in the United States soared by 3 million between 1996 and 2003, but the total population also grew. In fact, the proportion of the population that was uninsured remained the same: 15.6 percent. According to Census Bureau data, the fraction of Americans who report themselves uninsured, while varying from year to year, has been relatively constant over more than a decade, at about 15 percent.

Americans without Insurance

YEAR	PERCENTAGE
2003	15.6%
2002	15.2%
2001	14.6%
2000	14.0%
1999	14.3%
1998	16.3%
1997	16.1%
1996	15.6%
1995	15.4%
1994	15.2%
1993	15.3%
1992	15.0%
1991	14.1%

Source: Census Bureau

Myth 2: There are 46 million uninsured.

The number 46 million is accepted as a fact in political stump speeches, Hollywood movies, and Robin Cook novels. But as much as the estimate is repeated, it creates—in the words of Douglas Holtz-Eakin, director of the Congressional Budget Office—"an incomplete and potentially misleading picture."[7] Let's start by considering the source of that figure.

The Current Population Survey, conducted by the Census Bureau for the Bureau of Labor Statistics, looks at about 50,000 households. It's a thorough tool, but hardly without shortcomings. For one thing, the CPS does not consider the question of citizenship. Roughly 20 percent of the uninsured in this country are not citizens, which means the CPS finds that 36 million *Americans* lack insurance.[8] Immigration—legal and otherwise—skews the CPS numbers. (The difficulties faced by noncitizens are serious, but they speak to an immigration issue, not the failings of the health-care system.) The CPS also has problems, for instance, with the way respondents are asked to calculate the previous calendar year.[9]

Other surveys, like the Medical Expenditure Panel Survey (MEPS) and the Survey of Income and Program Participation (SIPP), have different approaches to sampling and find different results. In 2003, the Congressional Budget Office looked at the various studies that attempt to calculate the number of uninsured Americans.[10] Far from coming up with a single number, they found a staggering range:

- 21 to 31 million Americans were uninsured for the entire year.
- 39 to 42.6 million Americans were uninsured at any point in time.
- 56.8 to 59 million people were uninsured at some time during the year.

Why the inconsistency? The problem isn't just differences among the studies, it's also the subject itself. The number of uninsured Americans is constantly changing, making estimates of the size of this population effectively a moving target. David Henderson, who served as health economist for President Reagan's Council of Economic Advisers, explains:

> Many people believe that the 4[6] million uninsured people in the United States are the same people, year-in, year-out. That belief is false. Imagine that Eastman Kodak invented a camera that could take a collective picture of those 4[6] million people and still show the detail of each person's face. Let's say the camera takes a picture of those people and then takes a picture 5 months later of the 4[6] million people who are without health insurance. Question: What percent of the people in the first photo are also in the later photo? Answer: about 50 percent. In

other words, fully half of the people who lack health insurance at a given time have health insurance just 5 months later.

Why is insurance noncoverage so transient in time?

Because most jobs in the United States carry health insurance for those employees who want it and many of the non-insured are people who are out of work. Because unemployment is short-term for most people who are unemployed in a given year—the median duration of unemployment in 1998, for example, was 7 weeks—going without health insurance is also short-term.[11]

Both the Census Bureau and the CBO note the transient nature of noninsurance. Based on SIPP data from the 1990s, the Census Bureau suggests that the average family who loses coverage will become insured again in roughly 5.6 months.[12] Looking at the SIPP data, the CBO also calculated the duration of spells of noninsurance, and found that 84 percent of the uninsured are without coverage for less than 24 months.[13]

Uninsured Spells

DURATION OF NONINSURANCE	PERCENT
Under 4 months	45%
5 to 12 months	26%
13 to 24 months	13%
More than 24 months	16%

Source: CBO

Here is the underlying point: there are many gaps in coverage with an employer-based health-care system. The executive who leaves his corner office at Citigroup to look for greener pastures may soon join the ranks of the uninsured. His health hasn't changed; his insurability hasn't changed; only his employment status has. If this gentleman lands a vice presidency at a rival bank, we would consider this a success story. Yet, statistically speaking, he became part of the group of uninsured Americans. This example isn't simplistic; the crude statistic on the number of uninsured is.

Myth 3: The uninsured are a relatively homogeneous group— poor.

People assume that the uninsured are the poorest of Americans, a group that simply doesn't have the means to afford coverage. Many an episode of the television series *ER* turns on the predicament of the inner-city single mother, saddled with medical illness and three children, but lacking any insurance coverage.

Hollywood depictions notwithstanding, the single mom with three children is not uninsured—she has Medicaid, as do her children (and, for that matter, their neighbors). Who, then, are the 46 million? With little fanfare, the BlueCross BlueShield Association released "The Uninsured in America," a report that sheds light on the issue, in part by carefully analyzing the Census Bureau data.[14]

The BlueCross BlueShield report comments on the great heterogeneity of the uninsured. In all, roughly one-third of those households lacking insurance earn at least $50,000 a year. Now, depending on family size and location, $50,000 may not be an enormous sum of money; but that income level is certainly far above the poverty line. Most remarkably, this is the fastest-growing group among the uninsured (see table, page 88). A full 16 percent, the study notes, have incomes above $75,000 a year. "The Uninsured in America" also estimates that as many as one in three of the uninsured are eligible for government-sponsored health programs, but have not signed up.

That still leaves millions of people without insurance. Here too, the study finds a variety of situations. Around 6 million Americans lack insurance for only a few months. The chronically uninsured, the report suggests, number about 8.2 million.

Many Americans are uninsured by choice. Some of these are eligible for Medicaid, but choose not to sign up. Given that any hospital in America allows a Medicaid-eligible patient to do the paperwork right in the ER, there are few dire consequences to this type of lack of insurance. Recall, too, that about one-third of those without coverage earn more than $50,000 a year. Outside of a tiny minority that suffers from chronic illness, these people could afford coverage, but opt not to have it. This group, relatively well off yet uninsured, is particularly interesting. Consider that these individuals are at great risk of financial loss—a heart attack may result in bills amounting to tens of thousands of dollars. Why do they opt to go without insurance?

A study done by the California Healthcare Foundation looks at the nonpoor uninsured in the nation's most populous state.[15] This study uses a basic criterion: income that is twice the poverty level (a larger group than the $50,000+ income criterion). The group is not necessarily affluent: more than one-third had annual household incomes below $30,000, and only 10 percent had household incomes of $75,000 or more. Nonetheless, 40 percent of the sample reported owning their homes, and more than half had a personal computer. Why the lack of insurance? One clue is that 60 percent reported being in excellent or very good health, and 46 percent had not seen a health professional—even a chiropractor or an acupuncturist—in the previous year. The mean annual health expenditure was $200.[16] Not surprisingly, a majority (57 percent) of respondents *disagreed* with the statement, "Health insurance ranks very high on my list of priorities for where to spend my money."

Change in the Uninsured by Household Income, 1993–2003

INCOME	PERCENT CHANGE
< $25,000	–15%
$25,000 to $50,000	13%
$50,000 to $75,000	54%
$75,000+	130%

Source: Census Bureau

Myth 4: Health insurance equals health service—if you lack the former, you can't get the latter.

Many argue that the uninsured simply fall through the cracks, assuming that a lack of health insurance is the same as a lack of health care. "If you ain't got no money, you get a band-aid, a foot in the ass, and you're out the door," according to Denzel Washington in the movie *John Q.* In this view, there is no safety net.

Yet billions of dollars a year are spent on health care for the uninsured. In a study published by *Health Affairs,* Jack Hadley and John Holahan, both of the Urban Institute, look at the care received by the uninsured.[17] Using government data from 2001, they consider out-of-pocket spending as well as public and private contributions.[18] Hadley and Holahan peg the total amount of money spent at $98.9 billion a year.

Let's put that number in perspective: per person, the health care of the uninsured costs $1,587 a year.[19] By comparison, those with private insurance spend about $2,484 a year. Thus, there is a gap; but "no coverage" clearly is not synonymous with "no care." As Hadley and Holahan point out, significant amounts of money are spent by and for the uninsured, and only a small portion of this actually comes from their own pockets—just one of every four dollars. The rest comes from a variety of sources, including workers' compensation, free clinics, and direct Medicaid. There is another $34.5 billion of "uncompensated care," that is, care not paid for either out of pocket or by a private or public insurance source. This amount represents 35 percent of the cost of care for the uninsured. Hadley and Holahan found that most of this is actually covered by government expenditure:

> We also estimated that governments finance most of the uncompensated care received by the uninsured, spending about $30.6 billion on payments and programs largely justified to serve the uninsured and covering possibly as much as 80–85 percent of uncompensated-care costs through a maze of grants, direct provision programs, tax appropriations, and Medicare and Medicaid payment add ons. Most of this money comes from the federal government, primarily through Medicare and Medicaid, followed by state/local tax appropriations for hospitals, Medicaid DSH and UPL payments, and the VA's direct care programs.[20]

In all, then, governments spend about $30.6 billion annually on care for the uninsured, but in a round-about, heavily bureaucratic manner. There is also another $13.8 billion of cost that gets picked up by public programs. That is, rather than direct funding for care of the uninsured, there is a labyrinth of programs. (We'll return to this point shortly.)

Myth 5: 18,000 people die every year because they lack insurance.

Few organizations have as much prestige as the Institute of Medicine. Chartered by Congress, it has a governing council that reads like a Who's Who of the medical world—deans, university presidents and vice presidents, the editor of the *Journal of the American Medical Association,* and a former cabinet secretary. So when the Institute of Medicine declared that "About 18,000 unnecessary deaths occur each year because of lack of health insurance,"[21] the statistic gained immediate credibility. Besides, it makes sense that lacking insurance would affect use of the health-care system and thus health outcomes.

But the institute's number doesn't reflect the result of a study. In fact, their original report on the uninsured didn't mention the figure. It was only later, when the organization called for universal health care, that they decided to provide an "estimate."[22] The number 18,000 is based on various small studies suggesting poorer clinical outcomes when people lack insurance.

Most of these studies are not clear-cut. Consider, for instance, the landmark study on breast cancer outcomes in relation to insurance status. Dr. John Ayanian, an internist affiliated with Harvard, and his co-authors found lower survival rates for those lacking insurance. Their paper, published in the *New England Journal of Medicine,* is widely quoted. But here's the catch: Dr. Ayanian found even lower survival rates for those with Medicaid. In other words, if lack of insurance can be argued to have a negative effect on health, Medicaid coverage is worse. Taking their conclusion a step further, it would seem that the nation's poor would do better if we scrapped Medicaid.

Other studies are equally unsatisfying. Health outcomes are influenced by complex variables, such as socioeconomic status, but almost none of the commonly quoted studies make the necessary adjustments.

If myths surround the topic of the uninsured, are American politicians nonetheless taking the right steps to help people obtain coverage?

HillaryCare at Work

That millions go chronically without insurance is a major issue in a health-care system filled with problems. These people are not the very poor (who are covered by Medicaid). Many are working poor. They have employment, but no insurance because of its high cost. In some ways, of course, they *are* covered. In the event of a disaster, they can find care in the emergency rooms of America. They are thus covered for heart attacks, car accidents, strokes, and the like. The care will be excellent and, for the most part, free—the expenses are written off, or perhaps hidden in the bills of those who have insurance. But when it comes to basic primary and preventive care, too many go without.

Insurance is expensive. For middle-class Americans, though, paying a few thousand dollars isn't an obstacle. But what of the waitress who earns $15,000 a year? Or the freelance writer, fresh from college, who barely makes $17,000? State governments could work to ensure that less expensive insurance is available, but instead they have done the opposite. *Iatrogenic* is the term that doctors use to describe the phenomenon of medical intervention *causing* the patient's problem. Likewise, politicians craft policies that end up hurting the very people they aim to help. David Frum of the American Enterprise Institute provides some analogies:

> Suppose America's working poor were having terrible difficulty affording clothes. It would hardly make sense to pass a law compelling them to shop only at Neiman Marcus or Saks Fifth Avenue. Suppose car prices were rising fast. Who would propose outlawing the sale of used cars?[23]

Yet that is essentially what state governments have done in the arena of health insurance.

"IT WAS ONE YEAR FROM euphoria to defeat," writes Paul Starr at the beginning of his lengthy essay on the rise and fall of President and Mrs. Clinton's grand plan to remake American health care.[24] Prof. Starr, a Princeton sociologist and White House adviser,

observes that in September 1993, the president's pollster suggested that two-thirds of Americans supported the plan. Major
organizations like the American Medical Association embraced
universal coverage. In all, twenty-three Republican senators signed
on to full insurance. After a year, however, nothing remained. So
the story is told by Starr and others. But it omits one detail: at
the state level, it was not all a loss.

HillaryCare embodied the enthusiasm of the time for government intervention. While the White House failed in its grand
designs, many states forged ahead with a similar prescription.
Howard Dean's Vermont would be a good example of this. After
his governorship, Dr. Dean went on to run for president. Many
supporters cited his record on health care as proof of his successful leadership.

Vermont would hardly seem to be a likely candidate for
aggressive government intervention. According to the Census
Bureau, only 9.5 percent of Vermont's population lacked insurance when Dean assumed office in 1991. But HillaryCare was in
the air. "Every governor has his obsession," notes John
McClaughry, a former state senator who runs the free-market
Ethan Allen Institute.[25] "Health care was his. He worked on it until
he lost sight of the big picture."

First, Governor Dean meddled in the private insurance market. Before his swearing-in, Vermont's legislature passed a bill
mandating "community rating" and "guaranteed issue" for health
insurance. "Community rating" means that premiums are not
based on age or health status. Its purpose is to reduce premiums
for the chronically ill. "Guaranteed issue" requires insurance companies to sell policies to all applicants. Again, the aim is to improve
access for those who aren't healthy.

While these mandates may appear innocuous in and of themselves, in combination they create perverse incentives for people to game the system. People can buy insurance *after* they get
sick—and yet they still pay the same rates as other people their
age. A downward spiral for private insurers follows. Faced with
massive rate hikes, small employers drop coverage, often affect-
ing young workers disproportionately. With an insurance pool of
older and sicker workers, those left face high premiums.

One of Dean's first actions as governor was to champion Bill 160, a sweeping initiative to address the health-care problems he inherited. But instead of undoing the price regulation that had been slapped on the insurance industry, Bill 160 went further in the same direction. The legislation aimed to establish state control over hospital budgets, create a statewide insurance pool, and form a new health authority to coordinate it all. Instead of scrapping community rating, the legislation expanded it. Premiums wouldn't be based on age at all, but would be one-size-fits-all. Thus, a 20-year-old worker in perfect health would pay the same premium as a 60-year-old man with heart disease and emphysema. Much of the legislation was eventually dumped, but not community rating. "We fought that tooth and nail," recalls Tory Bunce of the Council for Affordable Health Insurance, an advocacy group for small businesses and insurance carriers. "We predicted that premiums would go through the roof."[26] They did.

If homeowners' insurance were regulated the way Governor Dean regulated health care, residents could insure their houses *after* they caught fire. As a result, healthy young people dropped their insurance; numerous insurance carriers left the state; and the percentage of uninsured Vermonters approached 14 percent.

Various ideas were floated in the mid-1990s to cope with the collapsing market for private health insurance. Some Vermont legislators proposed a single-payer plan. Dean's alternative was simply to expand government programs. In particular, he enlarged Medicaid, the federal-state program for poor Americans, with Washington footing most of the new cost. He expanded eligibility, going so far as to allow children in families with incomes up to $51,000 to be enrolled.

What does Vermont health care look like today? Insurance premiums are sky high. "I'm paying a lot and getting little choice," a self-employed Burlington resident told me. He wasn't kidding: To cover his wife and himself, he pays $5,000 a year for a plan with a $1,000 deductible. If that sounds like a stiff bill, it is. Frank Mazur, a Republican state representative, notes that "a high-deductible ($2,250) individual insurance policy for a 33-year-old in Vermont currently costs $215 a month. In New Hampshire, the policy costs $128 a month, and in South Carolina, $76 a month. Differences in population are a minor factor but community rating and guaranteed issue are major impediments to health insurance costs in Vermont compared to other states."[27]

Most carriers have left the state. There are only a few insurance companies open for business. At one time, thirty-three companies served the individual market. Today, there are two.[28]

Vermont, though, is hardly alone when it comes to experimenting with guaranteed-issue laws. Consider the sorry state of New Jersey's individual market.[29] In 1994, a New Jersey family policy (known as "Plan D") with a $500 deductible and a 20 percent copayment (i.e., the insurer pays 80 percent) cost between $504 and $1,076 a month. By January 2002, after the introduction of guaranteed issue, that same policy cost between $3,085 (Blue-Cross BlueShield) and $17,550 (Trustmark) per month. According to the Coalition Against Guaranteed Issue, it now costs more to buy family health insurance than it does to lease a Ferrari.

Ferrari versus New Jersey Insurance Costs

MONTHLY PREMIUM FOR A $500-DEDUCTIBLE FAMILY INSURANCE	
Aetna	$ 5,855
Celtic	$21,992
Fortis	$17,356
Guardian	$ 6,371
Guardian PPO	$ 6,556
Horizon BC/BS	$ 5,239
Oxford Health	**$ 3,780**
Trustmark	$20,393
United Health Care	$ 7,414
MONTHLY PAYMENT FOR A 2002 FERRARI 360 F-MODENA	
6-month lease	$2,523 to **$2,788**
48-month lease	$2,215 to $2,448
60-month lease	$2,023 to $2,236

Source: Coalition Against Guaranteed Issue

State regulation of private insurance isn't limited to insurance pricing rules like guaranteed issue. States across the country have also dictated which services and health-care providers must be covered. All insurance policies in Maine, for instance, must cover pastoral counseling. Maryland legislators thought it necessary to dictate how long a man stays in hospital after surgery for testicular cancer. These examples are hardly exceptional. In 1965, only seven benefits were mandated by the states; in 2004, according to the Council for Affordable Health Insurance, there are 1,823.[30] The list includes: acupuncturists (in 11 states), chiropodists (3), chiropractors (47), denturists (2), marriage therapists (4), massage therapists (4), osteopaths (24), and social workers (28). Some states also mandate that specific services be covered: birthing centers with midwives (6), breast reconstruction (48), clinical trials (19), dental anesthesia (27), hair prosthesis (7), IV fertilization (15), maternity stay (50), off-label drug use (37), second surgical opinions (11), and treatment of TMJ (temporomandibular joint) disorders (19).

Politically, these regulations reflect the power of lobby groups at the state level. Because large employers often self-insure and many of the above requirements exempt the small-group market, there isn't a counterbalance to the advocacy of, say, chiropractors. Add to the mix legislators eager to regulate fairness, and finding a simple insurance plan is a formidable task. Requiring coverage for a deluxe array of services inevitably raises premiums. Returning to David Frum's example, how much would clothing cost if the government required people to purchase it all from Saks and Neiman Marcus?

One of the leading online insurance brokerages, eHealth-Insurance, compared average insurance costs (for the individual market) among the states, drawing on data from 82,000 customers. Policies in New Jersey are triple the cost of those in Iowa.[31] (This comparison didn't adjust for age or type of coverage.) In a follow-up study, they compared the cost of a standard family insurance policy ($2,000 deductible with a 20 percent coinsurance) across the nation's 50 largest cities, involving some 4,000 insurance plans and 140 insurance companies.[32] The results are startling (see table, page 96). Consider: a non-employer-based family policy for four in Kansas City, Missouri, costs about $170 per month, while similar coverage in Boston tops more than $750 a month. Unpublished data on the small-group market—which serves smaller companies—also suggest great variability: similar HMO coverage for a business in New Jersey is one-third more per employee than in California.

Average Cost of Health Insurance by State
for eHealthInsurance Customers

STATE	AVG. ANNUAL PREMIUM
Iowa	$1,236
Ohio	$1,584
Connecticut	$2,088
New York	$3,540
New Jersey	$4,080

Monthly Premiums for Family Health Insurance by City

Kansas City, MO	$171.86
Long Beach, CA	$180.00
Tuscon, AZ	$184.88
Philadelphia, PA	$265.80
Chicago, IL	$359.01
Seattle, WA	$410.00
Minneapolis, MN	$529.00
New York, NY	$712.77
Boston, MA	$767.30

Source: eHealthInsurance

Not surprisingly, some businesses and individuals opt out of paying the stiff fee. In a study published in 1999, the Health Insurance Association of America suggests that one in four individuals without coverage are uninsured because of the high costs associated with state regulations. For all the attempts to make insurance fairer and more comprehensive, many people ended up joining the ranks of the uninsured.

What to Do?

A lack of results is often confused with a dearth of action. When it comes to health reform, the political rhetoric often echoes this mistaken conclusion—pundits and politicians speak of "finally" doing something for the uninsured. In the 1990s, HillaryCare collapsed, but massive state experiments carried on. States regulated what private insurance must cover and at what price; government programs like Medicaid were dramatically expanded. What was the result? More government, at more cost, but with little positive change.

In 2004, RAND Health released a summary of six major studies on the uninsured. "State Efforts to Insure the Uninsured: The Unfinished Story" considers the net effect of these efforts.[33] Despite the clear biases of the authors, none of the state initiatives—the regulations, government subsidies, and government expansions—appear to have addressed the problem of the uninsured. Indeed, despite the heavy spending, the only thing that has obviously changed is *who* provides coverage: public programs "crowd out" private insurance. (Undaunted by their own data, the authors conclude that "policymakers have learned valuable lessons," and they prescribe more of the same.)

Instead of pushing along the same lines, here's an alternative vision for helping the uninsured: first, make insurance options less expensive; second, help those who really need it.

First, Make Insurance Affordable

If we want more Americans to buy health coverage, we need to provide them with lower-cost options.

Health Savings Accounts. We need to entice people into the health insurance market. A low-cost option—exactly what HSAs represent—is a start. After all, health savings accounts move away from costly, all-inclusive coverage and toward lower-cost, catastrophic insurance. As noted in the last chapter, the economist Martin Feldstein observes that a typical Blue Cross of California family policy costs $8,460 annually (with a $500 deductible per member) compared with $3,936 for a similar HSA-style policy with a $2,500 deductible.[34] In other words, the HSA approach is a good deal.

But this isn't simply the observation of an economist. Look at the new HSA holders and we see the response of people to the marketplace: many of those establishing HSAs were previously uninsured. For the millions of middle-class Americans who have previously opted not to get insured, a more reasonably priced option may get them to put down the credit card and pick up the insurance card. It's encouraging that HSAs are now offered by every major insurance carrier.

Here is a subtle way of further enhancing the appeal of HSAs: increase the annual contribution cap. At present, the amount deposited in the health account cannot exceed the deductible of the catastrophic plan. But the cap means that a healthy young person—a group disproportionately represented in the ranks of the uninsured—may choose not to buy the plan. Raise the cap, and people will see HSAs as a long-term saving vehicle.

Out-of-State Insurance. Health savings accounts will take us only so far. In many states, like New Jersey and New York, state regulations have decimated the number of insurance carriers and driven up the cost of coverage. The people most affected are the working poor, since they have been priced out of their market.

It would be ideal if state legislatures undid the damage, allowing people to purchase a barebones plan, free of the regulations they had previously imposed. Some states have, if hesitantly, taken a step in this direction. New Hampshire repealed guaranteed issue; Maryland allows the uninsured to purchase a mandate-lite insurance; Colorado permits barebones plans. Unfortunately, these states have proven to be the exception rather than the rule. After all, the political forces that pushed for the regulations in the first place have not disappeared.

It's also true that health savings accounts have tempered some of the damage wreaked by mandate-happy legislatures. Small expenditures come directly from the HSA, meaning that individuals ultimately choose whether they go to, say, a naturopath—and pay for it out of their account.

But more needs to be done. Washington could address the regulation craze and champion a competitive market for health insurance by simply allowing people the option of buying insurance from other states. Americans can buy out-of-state mortgages and bank with financial institutions thousands of miles away. Why not allow people to find a low-regulation (and thus low-cost) state in which to buy their health insurance?

The federal McCarran-Ferguson Act of 1945 empowers states to regulate "the business of insurance." Interstate restrictions now leave many Americans at the mercy of a small number of local health insurance carriers. But nothing prevents Congress from permitting interstate insurance sales, an action consistent with the Constitution's commerce clause. Individuals and small businesses would then be able to shop around for a low-cost policy—an affirmation of free-market principles. Congressman John Shadegg has proposed a reasonable bill to give Americans more choices in health insurance; I testified in favor of it before Congress.[35] Because of opposition by some congressmen (largely from New York and New Jersey), the bill unfortunately died.

Tax Reform. Finally, Washington needs to address the tax inequity of the present system. While employer contributions to health insurance are nontaxable, individuals must pay in after-tax dollars. Like Canadian or Australian tourists in Manhattan, individuals attempting to pay their own health insurance discover that some dollars are less equal than others.

The inequity in the tax code could be corrected in one of two ways: drop the employer-based preference or expand it to include all health insurance purchases. Probably the former is better—why should health insurance be favored by the tax code?—but it may be impossible to accomplish in the present political environment. Leveling the tax field, then, is the way to go, at least ending the discrimination against the self-employed. John Cogan, a former deputy director of the Office of Management and Budget, along with co-authors Glenn Hubbard and Daniel Kessler, suggests that this would reduce the effective cost of premiums by roughly 30 percent.[36] (Further tax reform is discussed in the last chapter.)

Second, Help Those Who Need It

Different levels of government already spend almost $44 billion a year providing care to those who lack coverage. But these programs for the uninsured are bureaucratic and inefficient, creating incentives for hospitals and local governments to game figures in an attempt to help themselves more than their patients.

Obviously, $44 billion is not a small sum of money—especially given that many uninsured citizens either are eligible for government assistance or come from families with incomes over $50,000. If the money were targeted at those in need, it would go a long way toward paying for private insurance. The problem is that while the spending is largely done out of Washington, states (and counties) are on the front lines when it comes to programs for the uninsured. Washington can't design a program on its own.

Instead, Washington can do something better: get out of the business of micromanaging provision for the uninsured. The federal government should offer block funding to states and allow them to experiment with coverage options. Undoubtedly, some states will take the money and focus it on the people who need it most: the chronically uninsured. By excluding the higher-income uninsured, as well as those already eligible for assistance, a state-created voucher program could potentially offer more than $7,000 a person for coverage—enough to buy insurance in any state of the union. There are numerous practical issues to work out, of course, but this much is clear: for the relatively small but significant number of Americans who are in need, a large sum of money is already available.

What's needed is not a battery of new programs. Rather, we need to focus our efforts better. It's just this approach that can help reform America's fastest-growing public program: Medicaid.

SIX

Mills' Revenge: Medicaid

AT THE STROKE OF MIDNIGHT on January 1, 1994, Tennessee embarked on one of the most ambitious health-care experiments in American history. If necessity is the mother of invention, Tennessee had struggled with necessity for years—costs were spiraling up in the state Medicaid program, yet millions remained uninsured. Governor Ned McWherter had a sweeping vision: he would completely revamp Medicaid, massively expand eligibility (covering 800,000 uninsured already in its first day), improve prevention and wellness, and, while doing all this, save money.

His vision was to employ managed care, with the state operating like a giant HMO, providing health insurance to those who needed it and paying the premiums for those who couldn't afford it. If that seems ambitious, it was. The *New York Times* dedicated two front-page stories to the experiment.[1] A fawning essay in *Health Affairs* commented: "TennCare has reversed the central paradox of American health care: continuous increases in health care spending accompanied by an equally steady decline in the number of insured Americans."[2]

The Tennessee experience symbolizes the Medicaid zeal of the 1990s—and the reality of this decade with unsustainable costs and failed experiments. After much expansion, Medicaid has become an expensive and bureaucratic program, not just in Tennessee but everywhere. Nationally, the cost of Medicaid now rivals that of Medicare. Just as significantly, Medicaid is a dizzying mix of contradictions: it is at once generous and stingy;

expensive and cheap; expansive and narrow. Medicaid covers the long-term care needs of a wealthy New Yorker with a clever lawyer, yet provides mediocre compensation for physicians, so that an inner-city child with asthma will struggle to find a pediatrician. The program consumes more than $300 billion annually, but pays providers a fraction of what private insurance does. Finally, Medicaid covers middle-class children in Vermont but sets up obstacles that prevent the poor from getting needed medicines.

Medicaid—not unlike employer-sponsored health insurance—is paternalistic. Medicaid's intellectual groundwork was laid in the 1940s, a time when penicillin was cutting-edge. Just as employer-sponsored plans need modernizing, with devolution of decision making back to consumers, Medicaid reform must involve recipients in making choices.

A Formula for More

Medicare and Medicaid were birthed in the same bill, yet their histories couldn't be any more different. John Iglehart, editor of *Health Affairs,* has noted that after President Johnson's 1964 win, the creation of Medicare seemed "almost a foregone conclusion, although its final design reflected countless compromises." In contrast, Medicaid was "a child of Congress," an afterthought.[3]

Congressman Wilbur Mills, as chairman of the House Ways and Means Committee, added provisions for the program as part of his 1965 Medicare-creating legislation. Wilbur Cohen—who helped Mills draft the legislation and later served as secretary of Health, Education, and Welfare—later remarked: "Many people, since 1965, have called Medicaid the 'sleeper' in the legislation. Most people did not pay attention to that part of the bill. . . . [I]t was not a secret, but neither the press nor the health policy community paid any attention to it."[4]

For decades, Medicaid remained the poorer, smaller cousin of Medicare, covering only people on some form of welfare (Aid to Families with Dependent Children or Supplemental Security Income). The program's annual cost initially was under a billion dollars.[5] But as health expenses grew in the 1970s, Medicaid's budget steadily expanded. Medicaid is a public program with the same basic problem as private insurance: recipients hardly face any direct costs. A trip to the family doctor and an ER visit are largely free; if a state requires a copay, it would be only a dollar or two.

From the perspective of coverage, Medicaid is, in theory, the most generous health insurance. Since it covers prescription drugs and long-term care, it is broader in scope than Medicare. Unlike even the most elaborate private plans, Medicaid has neither a deductible nor a significant copay. There are reasons for such a financial arrangement. Yet the consequence is that Medicaid recipients have unfettered access to the most technologically sophisticated health-care system in the world—and therefore the cost of the program is high.

Further complicating the situation is Wilbur Mills' design: Medicaid is shared by two levels of government. The program is largely funded and regulated by Washington, yet administered at the state level.[6] To offset the disparities in wealth among states, the federal government contributes based on a formula, aiming to assist the less fortunate.[7]

In the early 1980s, the Reagan White House proposed a simple and elegant approach: convert Medicaid from an entitlement to a block grant. President Reagan's idea—which passed the Senate in 1982 with bipartisan support but was dropped from budget negotiations—would have left states with a fixed amount of money to spend as they saw fit.[8] With such a move, the administration hoped that state governments would rethink the program, reining in costs along the way.

But if the White House worried about budgetary restraint and contemplated financing, Congress saw Medicaid as a compassionate way to help the less affluent. In 1986, Congress loosened eligibility requirements. Medicaid's growth accelerated.

The resulting explosion in Medicaid spending relates directly to the program's structure. From a distance, the federal/state split seems to make sense: states have freedom to experiment, developing programs that best meet their needs. The basic funding formula also appears fair: Medicaid aims to help the less fortunate, regardless of geography. But together, these arrangements are disastrous because they leave states with great ability to re-engineer the program with someone else (Washington) footing the bill.

Rising Expenditures: Medicaid Spending from 1970

YEAR	EXPENDITURE IN BILLIONS
1970	$5 billion
1975	$13
1980	$26
1985	$41
1990	$73
1995	$156
2000	$207
2005	$330 (estimated)

Source: Centers for Medicare and Medicaid Services

Consider that the average federal contribution is 57 cents on every Medicaid dollar, meaning that an enterprising governor can offer his citizens new services without spending much from his state treasury. Historically, expanding Medicaid has been a good deal for the states. In fact, for every dollar of new state spending required for, say, a children's health program in West Virginia, Washington will pony up three "free" dollars.

With Washington eager to loosen eligibility requirements, states had a license to expand on the cheap. As Governor Bill Owens of Colorado explains, "it's a formula for more."[9] Needless to say, Medicaid's scope has expanded dramatically in recent years—the enrollment has nearly doubled since 1990—and this has been largely on Washington's dime. Once intended to serve only welfare recipients, the program now covers more than 50 million Americans.

Thus the great Medicaid expansions of states like Tennessee. Over a decade since its creation, TennCare seems more like a nightmare than the dream envisioned by Governor McWherter. Costs exploded, rising from $2.5 billion in 1995 to $8 billion in 2004. The program today consumes more than one-third of the state budget. Despite repeated efforts to tighten eligibility, it still covers 1.3 million of the state's 5.8 million people.

At least part of the problem is that TennCare was ripe for fraud and abuse. According to program audits, TennCare spent millions covering 14,000 dead enrollees. Another 16,500 enrollees lived out of state (some as far away as Hawaii). In fact, of 98,000 enrollees studied, 20 percent were found ineligible to be in the program. Amazingly, everyone seemed to abuse the program, even hundreds of state employees—who are eligible for the less encompassing state employee plan but not supposed to enroll in Medicaid.

But the larger problem is structural. Prescription drug costs alone increased more than 20 percent in 2005 alone, as there are effectively no limits on the drugs the system will pay for. When a family doctor prescribes aspirin, it's covered. So too are antacids, and a long list of other over-the-counter products.

In an unusual twist, reform efforts have been stymied by aggressive litigation. As the *Wall Street Journal* noted, "If TennCare denies a claim for a drug or any other type of care, an appeal can be filed for next to nothing. Fighting each appeal costs the state as much as $1,600 in legal fees. With 10,000 appeals filed every month, it's often easier and cheaper to pay a claim, regardless of the merits."[10]

Despite all the problems, does TennCare provide value for money? Sure it's expensive, but are recipients healthier for it? The evidence is mixed, at best. In 2001, Christopher Conover, an economist at Duke University, led a study comparing obstetrical care and birth outcomes in Tennessee and North Carolina. To that end, Conover analyzed data from over 300,000 birth records. He found almost negligible difference between Medicaid and Tenn-Care—in fact, Tennessee mothers were less likely to use prenatal care.[11] In a more thorough study for the Urban Institute, Conover looked at a variety of measures and a dozen papers considering quality—and again found the evidence of improvement mixed.[12]

TennCare has been the most sweeping experiment, but not the only one. In New York, Governor Mario Cuomo expanded Medicaid, turning New York City, one of the most prosperous cities in human history, into a Medicaid ghetto. After years of Governor George Pataki's abdication on this issue, New York still manages to spend more than California and Texas combined. Part of the heavy spending is because of provider reimbursement. But it's also true that New York offers generous Medicaid benefits. Recipients can get a month's supply of Viagra for just two dollars—a benefit that, until 2006, allowed incarcerated pedophiles to get the medication.[13]

Most states haven't been so bold, but they have still expanded Medicaid. Consider that states had the option of covering pregnant women up to 133 percent of the federal poverty level in 1990, but 31 states and the District of Columbia opted not to. Today, 35 states and the District of Columbia opt to cover pregnant women up to 185 percent of the poverty level.[14]

Medicaid spending has shot up by more than 60 percent in the last five years. Today, Medicaid's total budget rivals Medicare's, exceeding $300 billion, and it affects more Americans—some 50 million. The program's defenders are quick to suggest that Medicaid is needed by more Americans (a point we'll return to shortly). But if Medicaid covered only those Americans on some type of welfare, as it did historically, about 60 percent of today's recipients would be off the rolls.[15]

The program continues to swell. With no change in current law, the Congressional Budget Office projects, the cost will grow an average of 7.7 percent a year in the next decade. Governor Bob Taft of Ohio gave a speech entitled "Medicaid: The Monster in the Middle of the Road." He's not joking—nationally, state spending on Medicaid exceeds state spending on K-12 education.

At the end of 2004, the Bush administration floated—for the second time in two years—the idea of giving states more flexibility to administer the federal-state health insurance program for the needy, with a tradeoff: Washington would cap its contribution in the form of a block grant. "I think it would be a mistake to go down that road," said one senator. A governor opposed the idea "in any form." Another governor exclaimed at a press conference, "You don't pull feeding tubes from people. You don't pull the wheelchair out from under the child with muscular dystrophy."

All of these statements were made by Republicans. Senator Olympia Snowe of Maine warned the administration against change.[16] Mike Leavitt spoke against spending caps when he was governor of Utah a few years ago; now he's the secretary of Health and Human Services.[17] Governor Mike Huckabee of Arkansas worried about feeding tubes and wheelchairs being yanked away.[18]

Medicaid is in need of reform, but what have the governors done?

How *Not* to Reform Medicaid

States historically have been generous, and fiscal realities caught up. Faced with rising costs, every state has tried to find ways to stretch its Medicaid dollars. The biggest single idea to reform Medicaid: managed care. States hoped to find the solution for the increasing appetite of Wilbur Mills' program in the vision of Richard Nixon.

As with private insurance in the 1980s and 1990s, managed care has appealed to Medicaid administrators as a panacea—not only would they get spending under control, but Medicaid recipients could get better preventive care and chronic disease management. Medicaid managed-care enrollment jumped from under 12 percent of total enrollment in 1991 to 51 percent in 1999.[19] TennCare would be a case in point—a revamped program built on HMO coverage.

Managed care may be popular, but its efficacy at reining in costs is suspect. TennCare is a quagmire, with a series of recent governors battling to change the program, in part because of the fiscal disaster. And the managed-care experience outside of Tennessee has hardly been more inspired, according to Mark Duggan's research. An economist at the University of Maryland, he analyzed data from another hotbed of managed-care zeal, California, and concluded that not only did managed care actually *increase* costs, it brought no discernible change in health outcomes.[20]

Besides embracing HMOs, states have tried three other measures to get a handle on Medicaid spending: price controls, bureaucratic controls, and "creative" accounting.

1. States have cut or frozen reimbursement rates.

To save money, Medicaid underpays providers. Compared with private insurance and even Medicare, state governments' reimbursement is modest. In fact, for every dollar a physician collects for a service from Medicare, he or she will probably get 30 to 50 percent less from Medicaid for the same service.[21]

With so little pay, many physicians opt out, choosing not to treat Medicaid patients. According to a survey of physicians by the Medicare Payment Advisory Commission in 2002, only 39 percent were accepting all or some new patients (down from 48 percent a few years earlier).[22] A California physician explained his decision: "It cost me more to fill out all the paperwork than I can collect from MediCal." In one California study, a "Medicaid patient" contacted fifty orthopedic surgeons, and only three agreed to see him.

Speaking to the House Subcommittee on Health, Governor Jeb Bush of Florida described the serious problems facing Medicaid recipients:

> Consider that a child with cerebral palsy living in Volusia County must travel to Hillsborough County—a five-hour round trip—to see a neurologist and orthopedic surgeon to treat chronic back pain. Lack of local providers willing to participate in Medicaid reduces access to health care, and worse, perpetuates an inferior tier of care. This is only one example of the failures of the Medicaid program, but similar failures occur daily.[23]

Medicaid pays less than market rates for providers. That doesn't just affect providers who treat Medicaid patients; it affects everyone. Mark Duggan and Fiona Scott Morton (Yale) estimate that Medicaid increases the price of *non*-Medicaid prescriptions by 13 percent.[24]

2. States have created bureaucratic controls.

In an attempt to constrain spending, states have introduced a variety of rules and regulations. Nowhere is this more evident than with prescription drugs. Rather than allowing doctors to decide on prescription drugs for their patients, many states have implemented formularies—in effect, dictating what drugs doctors can prescribe and when. At last count, forty-four states either have a formulary or have plans to create one.[25] Some states have gone further, capping the number of prescriptions that patients can get.

"If you're a doctor trying to prescribe a non-formulary drug, prior approval means that you'll have to call a state agency and—most likely—wait on hold for up to 2 hours. How many doctors are going to do that?" asks Jim Frogue, who has studied Medicaid issues for several years and now works for the Center for Transforming Health Care.[26]

Peter Cunningham and a group from the Center for Studying Health System Change discussed the results of these regulations in a *Health Affairs* study: "From the perspective of Medicaid enrollees, states' efforts to contain the rising costs of prescription drugs are having negative effects on their access to prescription drugs." More troublesome is the population most affected: "That these access problems are particularly high for people with chronic conditions—which include a disproportionately high number of Medicaid enrollees—also suggests that there is unmet need for at least some essential medications."[27] In light of this paper, the conclusion of an earlier study comparing Medicaid and privately insured AIDS patients is unsurprising, if disconcerting: "The better outcomes associated with private insurance are attributable to the more restrictive prescription drug policies of Medicaid."[28]

3. States have become "creative" with their accounting.

With so many rules, there is opportunity for states to find loopholes to enhance their federal transfers, a process euphemistically called "creative accounting."

Carol Herrmann, who administers Medicaid in Alabama, told the *Wall Street Journal* that creative accounting "is exactly what all of us do when we do our income taxes every year: We look at the law and use the law to our advantage."[29] The schemes are relatively simple: since the federal government matches state spending, state governments just need to "increase" their spending. The county could send money to the state government, for instance, which promptly transfers the money right back to the localities—except bookkeepers continue to carry the funds on the balance sheets. "Whoever figures out the best loopholes wins," comments Tom Scully, former head of the Centers for Medicare and Medicaid Services.[30]

Creative accounting was pioneered by Pennsylvania in the early 1990s. David Feinberg, frustrated by a congressional decision restricting the use of Medicaid funding, decided to "think up something else." His idea was for the state to set up a money transfer from counties to the state that involved county-owned nursing homes—an idea worth $850 million a year to Pennsylvania. Feinberg took a job at a private lobbying firm and traveled the country teaching states how to enhance their federal match.

They learned their lessons well. Today, creative accounting is rampant. Consider that California probably enhances its federal match by nearly 9 percent a year.[31]

As with so much of health policy, these ideas don't belong to one party or another. Republicans and Democrats embrace the same strategies. It was a Democratic governor in Tennessee who turned the whole program over to managed care; GOP governors—often fond of free-market solutions—embrace drug formularies. The dominant ideology isn't liberal or conservative. It's paternalistic, attempting to micromanage Medicaid right down to the prescription pad sitting on the family doctor's desk.

Getting Serious about Medicaid Reform

If it were easy, it would have been done already; but Medicaid reform is no simple task. For one thing, Medicaid covers very different populations with different needs. An idea that could work for a poor but healthy man would not work for a severely disabled boy. In fact, the costliest recipients are also the least financially able. Glib solutions—give everyone a voucher or come up with high copayments—just will not work for everyone. There are, however, a few principles that can be applied: Medicaid needs to be more focused; choice is key; payment should be based on output, not input.

As heavy as the task may appear, there is historic precedent in the reform of another government program: welfare. Both Medicaid and the old Aid to Families with Dependent Children (AFDC) were created by Congress with lofty aims, but their modern realities aren't so grand. Their structures are comparable: both are entitlements; both have encouraged states to expand

the programs on Washington's dime; both see Washington holding the levers of centralized controls.[32]

Welfare was reformed. Can the same be done for Medicaid?

It's about Coverage, Not Government Coverage

So many people who study and write about Medicaid are obsessed
with the idea of public coverage. Indeed, much of the academic
writing on Medicaid suggests that program expansion has been
successful because enrollment rates have soared. Certainly, that's
one explanation for the growth in the program.

But it's also possible that by loosening eligibility requirements, states took over the job of insurance—that they "crowded
out" private coverage. This could happen for a couple of reasons:
it's possible that individuals opted for the lower premiums of a
public plan and employers dropped coverage knowing that their
employees could get Medicaid. After all, if we made food stamps
available to middle-class kids in Vermont, enrollment in that program would soar, too.

David Cutler of Harvard University and Jonathan Gruber of
the Massachusetts Institute of Technology were the first
researchers to estimate a crowding-out effect associated with
Medicaid expansions in an NBER Working Paper. Using data from
the Current Population Survey (CPS) from 1987 through 1992,
they studied children and women of childbearing age who were
eligible for Medicaid. Based on this analysis, Cutler and Gruber
concluded that approximately 50 percent of the increase in Medicaid coverage associated with the eligibility expansions was offset by a reduction in private insurance coverage—a crowding-out
rate of 50 percent.[33]

The key, then, is not to expand Medicaid for the sake of Medicaid. That seems to be as much about cost shifting (from the private to the public sector) as about enhancing coverage. Instead,
we can recognize a common goal: having more people covered—
publicly *or* privately—is worthwhile. To that end, we need to
think about the overall issue, not simply Medicaid reform. An
important step, thus, would be to make insurance as attractive
an option as possible. As mentioned in the previous chapter, government regulation of both the individual and the small-group

market has driven up the cost of insurance. Allowing individuals the option of getting less expensive health insurance by allowing out-of-state insurance purchases makes sense. It would mean that in good economic times, the burden on Medicaid would decrease as employers and individuals buy their own coverage.

End the Custody Battle

Since Medicaid isn't quite "owned" by either level of government, the incentives are all wrong—from the impetus for states to expand Medicaid, to the temptation to be "creative" with accounting. Any reform must address the federal/state quagmire. The smartest idea? Recognize that President Reagan was right—Washington should get out of the game entirely.

Of course, there are details to work out. Would the block grant simply be an extension of the present system? Would Congress take the opportunity to rejig the financing, developing a new formula for state support? The former—which was the essence of the Reagan proposal—would be relatively easy to implement, but would mean that funding inequities were frozen in place. Thus, New York would always get more federal funding per person than Mississippi. The latter—an approach championed by the Gingrich Republicans in 1995—could be very disruptive in the short term, but would ultimately be fairer.

Regardless of how the block grant is formulated, there would be two significant effects. First, since Washington would only fund the program (rather than fund and regulate), states would have greater freedom to innovate and experiment. Second, faced with greater financial consequences to their actions, the states would be more accountable. Nothing would stop an adventuresome young governor with his eye on a White House run from dramatically expanding Medicaid's scope—but he now would be required to find the money in his own treasury.

But while block grants make sense, they lack support among the governors.[34] "Even fiscal conservatives in the governor's houses are opposed to a block grant," comments Jim Frogue of the Center for Transforming Health Care.[35] Frogue notes the strange situation: At a time when states openly oppose federal intrusion in other areas, they lobby against a decrease in federal restrictions on administering Medicaid. But then, they have a vested interest: with funding effectively capped and Medicaid costs spiraling up, states would face a greater and greater burden. There is thus a Catch-22: Medicaid costs are going through the roof because the program is poorly structured, yet there is much hesitation on significantly restructuring the program because costs are rising so dramatically.

If the governors are less than enthused, many senators are too. So unpopular was the idea on the Hill that the Bush administration didn't even include it in the 2005 budget, after months of talking it up.[36] The White House, thus, didn't invest much in terms of political capital. A compromise seems easy, however: allow the block grant to grow at triple the inflation rate for the first seven years, a small amount of money compared with an unreformed Medicaid program.

If the program isn't converted to block grants, Washington can still help with reform—by getting out of the way. When states like South Carolina suggest sweeping reforms, Washington could offer a blanket waiver, allowing the state to opt out of all Medicaid regulations. Call it the Empowerment Waiver: any state that wants to reform Medicaid by empowering recipients will be given a free hand to do so.

Empower Recipients

There really isn't a single Medicaid program, but as many as there are states and territories. Still, the pattern is clear: many states cover nonemergency ambulance rides, brand-name prescription drugs (even when generics are available), and chiropractic services. Nelson Sabatini, Maryland's former secretary of Health and Mental Hygiene, observes that for the majority of families covered by Medicaid in his state, it would be less expensive to buy private insurance on their behalf.

Is this really surprising? Medicaid, after all, provides almost no financial incentives for its recipients to consider costs or alternative arrangements. This is why John Adams Hurson, a member of the Maryland House of Delegates and president of the National Conference of State Legislatures, commented:

I am a Democrat, a liberal Democrat, but we can't sustain the current Medicaid program. It's fiscal madness. It doesn't guarantee good care, and it's a budget buster. We need to instill a greater sense of personal responsibility so people understand that this care is not free.[37]

Personal responsibility is crucial, and also tricky. Still, many—in fact, most—recipients are healthy and not elderly. Some innovative ideas for dealing with this population have been considered at the state level, most notably in Florida and South Carolina. Just as Wisconsin once led the way on welfare, these two states may represent the future of Medicaid.

Florida's Medicaid is more comprehensive than many private plans. Such generosity comes at a price, though. For the past six years, Medicaid spending has climbed 13 percent annually and now soaks up about one-quarter of the state budget. Costs are expected to rise to 35 percent of state revenue in the next four years. As a result, Governor Bush proposes something innovative: getting his state out of the business of micromanaging Medicaid.

Under his plan, those eligible for Medicaid would qualify for a set, need-based amount of money. With this money, recipients could pick a plan among competing insurance company offerings—from more comprehensive coverage to less comprehensive but at a lower premium, with part of the money saved going to a recipient's flexible spending account for out-of-pocket medical expenses. In addition, the state would offer incentives in the form of better benefits to those who live healthier lives.

The contrast between Florida's approach and that of many other states couldn't be starker. At a time when state governments are developing more and more elaborate ways of controlling Medicaid, Jeb Bush envisions Tallahassee doing relatively little. Besides funding, Florida would ensure transparency of the private plans and counsel Medicaid recipients about their choices.

Governor Bush's plan means that recipients are given more choice, yet it reins in spending by increasing competition among insurance plans. It's an innovative approach that controls costs, particularly since it involves recipients more in their health decisions. "It's fiscally wise and pro-patient," says Jim Frogue.

Governor Bush sees Medicaid recipients being offered a menu of choices. His counterpart in South Carolina also wants choice instilled in the program. Governor Mark Sanford has good reason to think of reform: between 1999 and 2004, South Carolina's Medicaid program grew annually by about 11 percent; in the 2005 budget, health services will eat up about 34 percent of all revenue. Governor Sanford summarizes the problems well: "You give the consumer—once qualified—unlimited purchasing power for a product that someone else is paying for."[38] His solution: empowering Medicaid recipients with health dollars.

Under Governor Sanford's proposal, if a managed-care plan costs $2,000 for a typical family, the money could be converted into a plan similar to a health savings account. This would mean purchasing a high-deductible catastrophic policy for the family (say, at about $1,200) and then depositing the remaining money into a personal health account. Recipients would be given a debit card to access their account.

Because of the special needs of the Medicaid population, the accounts wouldn't quite function like private health savings accounts. The accounts might cover, say, a $10 copay for a visit to the family doctor or part of the cost of a diagnostic test. Preventive medicine—immunizations, blood-pressure screening, diabetes tests—would continue to be free. To the frugal health consumer, the program would offer two advantages. First, money from the accounts could be used to purchase additional services, like eye care. Second, the beneficiary, upon leaving Medicaid, could roll over a portion of the unused money to a private-sector health savings account.

Reforming Medicaid is no easy task. A small proportion of recipients use a large share of the budget. Nationally, the commonly quoted figure is that 20 percent of users cost 80 percent of Medicaid dollars. South Carolina officials suggest that their usage is even more lopsided, at 5 to 55. As a result, Governor Sanford is unlikely to solve all of Medicaid's woes in one proposal.

The Florida legislature clipped the wings of the Bush plan, allowing it to be carried out only as an experiment in two counties.

The South Carolina proposal, in contrast, nears final approval. Allowing Medicaid recipients ownership of their health care—the thrust of both proposals—makes fiscal sense. It also means that Washington can push for change without anyone having to contemplate pulling feeding tubes or yanking wheelchairs.

End Medicaid for Millionaires

Stephen Moses of the Center for Long-Term Care Financing makes an important observation. Do a Web search for "Medicaid estate planning," he suggests, and marvel at the number of hits—nearly 600,000. Welcome to one of the fastest-growing areas of legal practice: elder law. Crafty attorneys can help families get seniors onto Medicaid for long-term care.

That would not seem noteworthy. After all, Medicaid aims to cover nursing-home care for the poor. But "Medicaid estate planning" isn't about helping the least fortunate in society. Rather, its purpose is to preserve assets and thus inheritance of middle-class and wealthy families. How to do this while getting seniors into long-term care facilities? Get the taxpayer to pick up the tab—a practice so commonplace that Medicaid now functions like inheritance insurance. Consider that for every dollar spent privately on nursing-home care, the public coffers contribute four.

Every state has requirements for Medicaid eligibility. Potential recipients are required to calculate their assets—but Medicaid rules allow these individuals to exempt many things: cars, the home, housing renovations, investments in the family business, and term life insurance. Indeed, this creates an unusual circumstance. A Rhode Island man with, say, three Mercedes Benz cars and a large Newport mansion can still qualify for Medicaid. That may sound ridiculous and morally dubious—but it is completely legal. (When it was revealed that Carol Moseley-Braun, a Democrat from Illinois, had done "asset-shifting" to get her mother qualified for Medicaid, she still managed to win her Senate race in 1992.)

In fact, the situation is even more absurd than that. Since federal law prevents long-term care facilities from evicting residents if they switch to Medicaid, wealthy seniors can get into a private, high-quality facility for a year—then shift their assets and remain in the desirable home.[39] Stephen Moses explains how this is done: "Poor people don't have key money, so they end up in the least desirable 100%-Medicaid facilities, while the lawyers' clients occupy the scarcer Medicaid beds in nicer nursing homes."[40]

Medicaid pays for more and more long-term care. Since it does, the desire to be insured for the high cost of such care diminishes. In an NBER Working Paper, Prof. Jeffrey Brown and Prof. Amy Finkelstein argue that long-term care insurance is crowded out by the public program.[41] Given that the amount of money spent on long-term care is projected to triple over the next thirty-five years, there is urgent need to address this problem before it's too late.

First, we need to encourage people to invest in long-term care insurance. Partnership programs—started by Health and Human Services but hamstrung by Congress—are a step in the right direction. They allow people to draw down their insurance before the rest of their assets, meaning that their inheritance is spared. Not only that, but since purchasers have money on hand, they can tailor their long-term care to their exact needs—like home care.

Second, Congress and the states must tighten up eligibility requirements for Medicaid. It's one thing to argue that Medicaid should be available to everyone who falls on bad times; it's another to believe that Medicaid ought to be available to millionaires. Filling in the loopholes could be done easily. There are, of course, other creative approaches as well.[42]

Not all of the problems with long-term care will be solved by focusing benefits more on those in need. The present commitment to long-term care is the costliest single part of Medicaid. What can be done about it?

Again, the basic principle should be paying for outcome, not input. Prof. Michael Bond of Ohio State University observes that many states do the opposite. Ohio, for example, pays for long-term care beds, not patients. As a result, Ohio pays for 13,000 empty beds.[43] If states are going to provide long-term care, they ought to do it intelligently—determining the needs of the patients, then accepting bids from competing providers.

"Cash and Counseling" Makes Sense

Of all the people covered by Medicaid, the disabled present the most difficult problem from a policy perspective; they are chronically ill and costly. It might seem that the only way to assist them is through some paternalistic program. But that is an overreaching conclusion.

Many states now experiment with Cash and Counseling programs. The idea is simple: for specific Medicaid beneficiaries who receive personal-care services at their homes, the state gives cash allowances so they can buy those services. Patients, thus, have the ultimate control: which providers are chosen, when, and at what cost. Unspent moneys can accrue in the Medicaid beneficiary's account, and eventually be used for larger items (like lift chairs to assist with stairs). Jim Frogue notes the popularity of this program:

> Patient satisfaction rates with the program are astronomical. In Arkansas, 96 percent of patients would recommend the program to others. Additionally, 82 percent say the program has improved their lives and 65 percent say it has improved their lives "a great deal." In New Jersey, 97 percent of those surveyed would recommend the program. Similar rates of satisfaction have been reported in Florida.[44]

Cash and Counseling programs aren't necessarily immediate money savers. As Frogue remarks, the evidence at the state level suggests that costs tend to be higher in the initial year, though by year two, the program is cost-neutral. More difficult patients also pose a problem. If someone is too incapacitated to make basic decisions, how could that person be expected to shop around for care? These individuals might be beyond the scope of Cash and Counseling—or maybe not. One option is to authorize a family member or social worker to make care decisions.

Colorado would be a case in point with its CDAS program, Consumer-Directed Attendant Support, which gives severely disabled Medicaid recipients more control over their care, putting them in charge of their own health dollars. Participants are able to hire and fire their own caregivers, and to use the money for life-enhancing equipment. Patient satisfaction is high, as is quality of care—but not costs. Whereas Medicaid state budgets skyrocket, CDAS spending is 20 percent under budget. "Choice works," declares Governor Bill Owens.[45] In 2006, tens of thousands of Colorado's nondisabled Medicaid recipients will be eligible for an expanded version of CDAS. More than half the states are experimenting with similar initiatives.

APART FROM STATE EXPERIMENTS with Cash and Counseling programs, reform efforts have typically pushed along the old paternalistic lines. Given that costs have never been higher, it seems time to consider alternatives. The above recommendations would transform Medicaid, focusing the program but also devolving decisions to individuals.

Some will charge that such a plan would end Medicaid as we know it. Linda Storey, who has battled multiple sclerosis for thirty-five years, would probably be in favor of just that outcome. An early enrollee in Colorado's CDAS, she commented: "It gives you your life back. I'm in control of my health now."[46]

Devolving decisions to individuals would transform Medicaid. It is also the key to changing the other Great Society healthcare program: Medicare.

SEVEN

Mills' Revenge II: Medicare

IF THE PRESIDENT OF THE UNITED STATES seemed tired on the afternoon of December 8, 2003, he had reason to be. Throughout the year, George W. Bush and his staff had spearheaded an effort to add a drug benefit to Medicare. To that end, they pulled together a remarkable coalition of unlikely bedfellows: big business, previously ambivalent about Medicare; big pharma, previously ambivalent about a Medicare drug benefit; and the AARP, previously ambivalent about a Medicare drug benefit proposed by Republicans. The work was not easy, with criticism from conservatives (who feared that the legislation went too far) and liberals (who fretted that it didn't go far enough).

But on December 8, the president claimed his prize. With the stroke of a pen, he substantially realigned Medicare, achieving a goal that had eluded his predecessor. But the real winner wasn't a president who took a Democratic issue and put a Republican stamp on it, thereby bolstering his re-election campaign the following year, but a man who had retired from Congress three decades earlier: Wilbur Mills.

Back in the 1960s, Mills had used his position as chairman of the House Ways and Means Committee to champion a federal health program for the elderly—over opposition from, among others, conservative Republicans. Jump ahead four decades, and a conservative Republican president was not only swearing by the compassion of the program, he was busy expanding it. The

Medicare Modernization Act of 2003 thus stands as the high-water mark for Medicare's political support.

Except that, in so many ways, the program is dying under its own weight. Despite the Great Society nostalgia of that day, Medicare as we know it is coming to an end. Let's be clear: the program remains popular and not a single prominent politician in America will do anything but lavishly praise it. And the purpose of the program—to provide health care to elderly Americans—has not become irrelevant. Yet Medicare, at just forty, has entered into its twilight because its basic financial assumptions have proven false. With spiraling per capita costs and a sea of new beneficiaries about to join the program, Medicare wilts.

The crisis in Medicare isn't solely financial; it's also structural. Medicare is fundamentally flawed, largely divorcing recipients from the financial consequences of their actions. The end result is an expensive and bureaucratic program that, in the long run, poses more of a financial disaster for the nation than Social Security.

After the exhaustive battles of 2003, it would be easy to conclude that Medicare can't be meaningfully changed. But the program will change—it's only a matter of time. Encouragingly, the first major step on the path toward a more sensible program has already been taken. Back in the late 1990s, Senator John Breaux and Congressman Bill Thomas issued a report on instilling Medicare with competition and choice. Their model for reform was simple enough: the health plan used by members of Congress and about eight million others.

In this chapter, we outline how such a system would work for Medicare.

Medicare Modernization Act

As Congress prepared to vote in November 2003 on the prescription drug benefit, many were enthusiastic. It wasn't just that Medicare was about to undergo its largest change in forty years; it was going to be a *Republican* change. The *Washington Times* editorialized that this legislation would help cement the GOP as the majority party. Tom DeLay, the House majority leader at the time, opined that the Medicare legislation "represents not only a new chapter in American health care but also a historic opportunity to put a conservative imprint on a major entitlement program in need of reform."[1] Other prominent Republicans agreed.[2]

But the prescription drug benefit is bad medicine for Medicare. Even if the legislation serves the short-term political interests of Republicans, it will create policy and political trouble for both parties in the coming years because it fails to address the fundamental issues with the program.

What's wrong with the Medicare Modernization Act? With apologies to Elizabeth Barrett Browning, let me count the ways:

1. *It's a massive solution to a small problem.* A full 76 percent of American seniors already had some type of prescription drug coverage. Of those without coverage, only a minority had minimal income (under double the poverty level) and maximal drug expenses (greater than $4,000 a year). In all, just 2 percent of seniors fell into this high-need category.[3] That's far too many Americans, but it doesn't justify the largest single expansion of a federal entitlement in three decades. Like trying to kill a mosquito with a machine gun, the approach is heavy-handed.

2. *It's the money, stupid.* Since Congress hopes to offer something for everyone, the program is slated to cost $400 billion over ten years. Incidentally, the National Center for Policy Analysis estimates that just one in every sixteen dollars will go to help low-income American seniors purchase drugs that they presently cannot afford.

3. *It misses the big issue.* The costs associated with Medicare will grow dramatically over the coming decades as our population ages. Far from correcting this unsustainable situation, a prescription drug benefit will significantly increase the liability—like planning to add a sauna and a gazebo to a house with a sinking foundation.

4. *There aren't any meaningful market reforms.* Instead of a sweeping new vision for the program, the Medicare Modernization Act promises only a demonstration program limited to a handful of urban centers and beginning in 2010. Former House majority leader Dick Armey observes: "I was in Congress long enough to know how demonstration projects really work. . . . On meaningful

needed reforms, demonstration projects mean a quiet, obscure death."[4] There is no shortage of dead demonstrations that could be cited, including the last set of Medicare competition projects.

5. *The drug benefit will inevitably expand.* Republicans enthuse that they've just stolen a liberal issue and made it their own. That may prove overly optimistic. Because of the "donut hole" in coverage—drug costs between $2,250 and $3,600 are borne by the individual[5]—politicians in the future will be tempted, in the words of Milton Friedman, to "fill in that hole."[6]

6. *It will lead to price controls.* With passage of this bill, the federal government will become the largest funder of prescription drug purchases in the world. Medicare already has price controls for physician fees and hospital reimbursements. Will it be long before Washington wants a better deal on pharmaceuticals?

There is one good thing buried deep in the Medicare bill: the creation of health savings accounts. But as far as Medicare reform goes, the Medicare Modernization Act fails to live up to its name.

How then to reform Medicare properly? Let's start by better understanding the program's problems.

The Four I's of Medicare

"Do you want to know why the Yankees always win?" asks the con man in *Catch Me If You Can.* When the FBI agent replies that it's because they've got Mickey Mantle, the con man offers: "No. It's because the other team's too busy staring at the pin stripes." For the past few years, the debate over Medicare's future has focused on the dazzling and the obvious: the Republican proposal to add a prescription drug benefit. The real issue, though, is subtler and has been lost from view: the structural problems of Medicare. On this score, Congress hasn't really begun to reconsider the Great Society program.

As noted above, if Medicaid was the accidental program, Medicare was the end result of decades of deliberation, debates, and votes—a historical inevitability, as some academics describe it. But the form and structure of Medicare was due to one man: Wilbur Mills.

As noted earlier, a major expansion of government into health care had been weighed since FDR's administration. By the late 1950s, Democrats focused on a smaller goal: health insurance for seniors. John F. Kennedy campaigned for president on the idea, promising to tie it to Social Security. President Johnson hoped to convert the campaign pledge into law but was stalled by the House Ways and Means Committee chairman, Wilbur Mills.

But Mills had a change of heart (perhaps influenced by his own presidential ambitions) and soon championed not simply hospital insurance, but also coverage for doctors. He persuaded the White House to turn around draft legislation overnight and then took the bill to committee. He managed to get Republican support—Wilbur Cohen described it as the greatest legislative maneuver he'd ever seen.[7]

Add up the outlays for Medicare and Medicaid, and they well exceed federal spending on Social Security and even defense. Wilbur Mills may not be a household name, but his efforts affect every household in America.

The Mills Influence: Government Spending in 2004 (in billions)

Medicare	$297
Medicaid	$309
Medicare + Medicaid	$606
Social Security	$492
National Defense	$454

Source: *Healthy Competition,* based on CBO numbers

Medicare is a program designed for the circumstances of its day. Mills' legislation was crafted at a time when the population was young; the number of elderly, relatively small; and the cost of medicine, minimal. A generous program, free at the point of care, seemed to make sense. But today, the high-tech, high-expense medical revolution has transformed care—and costs. When Medicare was created, officials projected that the hospital insurance would cost $9 billion in 1990. In fact, it cost more than seven times that amount.

The 2005 report of Medicare and Social Security Trust Funds is unequivocal in describing the difficulties facing the program:

Total Medicare expenditures were $309 billion in 2004 and are expected to increase in future years at a faster pace than either workers' earnings or the economy overall. As a percentage of GDP, expenditures are projected to increase from 2.6 percent currently to 13.6 percent by 2079 (based on our intermediate set of assumptions). The level of Medicare expenditures is expected to exceed that for Social Security in 2024 and, by 2079, to represent almost twice the cost of Social Security. Growth of this magnitude, if realized, would place a substantially greater strain on the nation's workers, Medicare beneficiaries, and the Federal Budget.[8]

Under current law, Medicare will consume 25 percent of federal income-tax revenues by 2030. In other words, Medicare threatens to be the program that ate the budget. The unfunded liability of Medicare—that is, how much the program will cost beyond what it will take in through payroll taxes and premiums for the next seventy-five years—is $68.3 trillion, or more than five times the present GDP of the United States.

Insolvency is thus Medicare's biggest single problem. Say what you want about the program's compassion; its bottom line is formidable. But Medicare's problems don't end there. Robert Reischauer, a former director of the Congressional Budget Office and the president of the Urban Institute, suggests that the problems are four I's: "Medicare is *inadequate, inefficient, inequitable* and it's *insolvent.*"[9]

Inadequate

Medicare covers many small bills yet leaves the elderly exposed to potentially enormous out-of-pocket expenses. Medicare thus violates almost all principles of sound insurance. Jesse Hixson, the retired principal economist of the American Medical Association, once calculated that seniors could be left on the hook for $35,000 under Medicare. While that amount is exceptional and rare, large expenditures are not. Every year, more than three-quarters of Medicare recipients pay $5,000 or more out of pocket.

Not surprisingly, most seniors have supplementary insurance, purchased either individually or by their former employers. These "Medigap" policies effectively fill in the coverage lacunae.

Much is written about the equality of Medicare—it covers all seniors, regardless of income. But this is deceptive. Health care for the elderly in America is really two-tiered: there is the standard, government coverage, and the coverage available to people with supplemental policies.

Inefficient

We could go further with the critique: Medicare is not really an insurance, since it doesn't cover catastrophic care or many pharmaceuticals (even with the expansion) or preventive care—all standard coverage in any private health plan. But Medicare does cover much and does so with limited direct cost to the patient. Further complicating the situation is a congressional requirement that Medigap policies be largely free of copays and deductibles.

Medicare, thus, has similar problems to private coverage: people are overinsured for the services that are covered. The *New York Times* describes one of the results in a front-page story:

> It is lunchtime, and the door to Boca Urology's office is locked. But outside, patients are milling about, calling the office on their cellphones, hoping the receptionist will let them in. To say they are eager hardly does them justice.
>
> "We never used to lock the door at lunch, but they came in an hour early," said Ellie Fertel, the office manager.
>
> "It's like they're waiting for a concert. Sometimes we forget to lock the door and they come in and sit in the dark."

One of the practice's urologists suggests that few of these patients have serious medical problems. The *Times* explains:

> Doctor visits have become a social activity in this place of palm trees and gated retirement communities. Many patients have 8, 10 or 12 specialists and visit one or more of them most days of the week. They bring their spouses and plan their days around their appointments, going out to eat or shopping while they are in the area. They know what they want; they choose specialists for every body part. And every visit, every procedure is covered by Medicare, the federal health insurance program for the elderly.[10]

Earlier, we considered the work of the Dartmouth Medical School researchers who looked at regional variations in care. Data at the hospital level also raise questions. Investigators recently released a paper evaluating care at hospitals leading *U.S. News & World Report*'s 2001 rankings for geriatric care, supposedly the best in America.[11] They found striking variations in the amount of care provided, with no association between higher intensity of interventions and better outcomes. (For instance, Medicare patients at Mount Sinai Medical Center in New York City during the last six months of their lives were in hospital twice as many days as Mayo Clinic patients.) Another paper from the Dartmouth group found that academic medical centers differed by up to 60 percent in the overall "intensity" of medical services offered to Medicare patients who had heart attacks, hip fractures, or colorectal cancer. Yet high-intensity care actually resulted in *worse* health outcomes.[12]

Drawing on such work, Elliott Fisher and co-authors estimate that "nearly 20 percent of total Medicare expenditures ... appears to provide no benefit in terms of survival, nor is it likely that this extra spending improves the quality of life."[13]

If Medicare seems indifferent to cost, what about quality? Palm Beach Gardens Medical Center in Florida suggests that this area is equally problematic. According to a lengthy *Washington Post* story, many—including the state inspectors—believed that the heart surgery unit was plagued with high postoperative infection rates. And there was an obvious reason. The place was a mess: "Dust and dirt covered some surgical equipment. Trash cans and soiled linens were stored in hallways. IV pumps were spattered with dried blood. One patient's wife said she saw a medical assistant tear surgical tape with his teeth."[14] How did Medicare deal with Palm Beach Gardens? It paid the trouble-plagued hospital more. After all, Medicare reimbursement is based on services provided. More infections mean longer hospital stays, more procedures and tests, and more money. Medicare isn't designed to reward performance or manage chronic disease.

Inequitable

Robert Reischauer's final point is one that has already been made here: there are enormous geographic variations in the program. A Medicare recipient in one state may cost a fraction of what another state's recipient costs the Treasury. Consider that in Hawaii, the average expenditure per year is $3,800; over in Louisiana, it's $6,700; and in Washington, D.C., it's $7,200 a year.[15]

Inequitable and inefficient combine for interesting and unpredictable results. In Oregon and Montana, for example, back surgeries are two to four times more common than in New York and New Jersey. It's possible to go a step further, looking at quality and expenditures on the state level. The Centers for Medicare and Medicaid Services (CMS) ranks quality of care based on crude indicators, like how many heart attack patients get an aspirin (the standard of care). As the following graph shows, the states with the most expensive care aren't necessarily besting the field in quality.

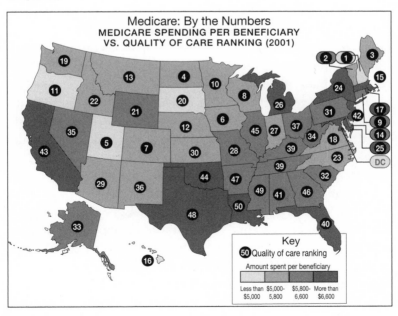

Medicare, in other words, is ripe for reform. But are we actually moving in the right direction?

How *Not* to Reform Medicare

On the one occasion I chatted briefly with Tom Scully in the White House basement, he appeared to be stressed. He had much on his plate: as administrator of the Centers for Medicare and Medicaid Services, he was essentially the single largest purchaser of health care in the country. Scully held that position for almost two years—to the frustration of many. Why the controversy? He explained his philosophy to the *Wall Street Journal,* likening his job overseeing federal health insurance for the elderly and the disabled to the carnival game whack-a-mole: "When spending shoots up, you whack it down."[16] Indeed, Scully had no difficulty making hard decisions about what procedures and drugs should be covered, and at what price. "We do the best we can to figure out the price we should pay, and that makes some people unhappy."[17]

Herein lies the problem: Medicare costs are climbing year after year. With little direct cost to the consumer, American seniors are overinsured. How then to rein in expenditures? The biggest single reform of Medicare historically—whether it be in Republican or Democratic administrations—has been the use of wage and price controls, combined with rigid regulations. As columnist Matt Miller once quipped, "There's the Kremlin-style central pricing, which once left Florida hospitals flooded with MRIs (by over-reimbursing for the machines after actual costs had dropped), while giving anesthesiologists (paid by the hour) a stake in keeping you under."[18]

Here are the results of Medicare central planning:

Poor physician participation. Many doctors hesitate to take new Medicare patients. In some places, such as Denver, it's hard for the elderly to find a doctor. Nationally, according to a new study by the Center for Studying Health System Change, nearly 30 percent of American physicians will not accept some or all prospective new Medicare patients.[19]

Regulatory excess. Medicare requires hospitals and other providers to comply with over 130,000 pages of regulations, according to a Mayo Clinic estimate.[20] A study for the American Hospital Association found that for every hour of care delivered to a Medicare patient, hospital officials spend roughly half an hour completing paperwork.[21]

Uneven service. As a government report on competition observes: "One unintended consequence of [Medicare's] administered pricing systems has been to make some hospital services extraordinarily lucrative and others unprofitable. As a result, some services are more available (and others less available) than they would be in a competitive market."[22]

Tom Scully summarizes the situation:

> In the long run, government price fixing for services has never worked in any system in any society, and I don't think that it can work here, either. Having federal price fixing, no consumer information or price sensitivity, and no measurement of quality has led to predictable results: artificially high prices and uneven quality.[23]

Scully left CMS in 2004; his experience there would be an example. He doesn't much believe in Medicare's central planning, but as administrator of CMS, he felt he should do it as well as possible—being the best wage and price controller around.

With baby boomers set to retire and start using Medicare, can the program just continue with its system of price controls? Robert Moffit, director of the Center for Health Policy Studies and a former official at Health and Human Services, answered this question in testimony before the Senate:

> The proposition that the government can control the growth in Medicare spending through the imposition of price controls or caps on overall Medicare spending is an intellectually unimpressive one; of course it can. But, likewise, there is no reason to believe that Congress can impose such controls and cap such spending and simultaneously accommodate the rising demand for those services without reducing their quantity or compromising their quality.[24]

There was a brief flirtation with an alternative in the late 1990s. When the Republicans won Congress, they attempted to tackle Medicare's spiraling costs. After much negotiation with the White House, they agreed to take on Mills' program with

Nixon's core idea: managed care. Since 1985, Medicare allowed seniors to voluntarily join a private managed-care health plan, but a limited number did so. Republicans sought to change this— and the entire Great Society program. As part of the Balanced Budget Act of 1997, Congress approved Medicare + Choice, giving seniors the option of a managed-care plan in place of traditional Medicare.

Since the days of the Nixon White House, the arguments forwarded have been the same: managed care would contain costs yet grant beneficiaries more choices and benefits. As a historical aside, before President Nixon touted managed care for employer-sponsored health insurance, he embraced the idea of converting Medicare over to managed care. If it was Nixon Republicans who had pondered such Medicare reform, the Gingrich Republicans would make it happen.

In its first years, Medicare + Choice seemed promising: enrollment in Medicare managed care swelled by almost 50 percent and a sea of HMOs competed for the business. But the honeymoon soon ended and divorce quickly followed: weighed down by low reimbursement rates, spiraling costs, and poor planning, HMOs pulled back. The number of participating plans fell. By 2002, enrollment had sunk to pre–Medicare + Choice levels.

This begs a simple question: isn't there a better way to reform Medicare, moving beyond Mills and Nixon?

What Your Mailman Knows

It's easy to summarize the chaos: a program that pushes toward insolvency; a demand for more far-reaching drug coverage and yet hesitation at its cost; a partisan split on how to address these issues. That was 1998, when a handful of politicians led by Senator John Breaux and Congressman Bill Thomas managed to achieve the impossible—a sensible plan to reform Medicare that enjoyed bipartisan approval. The secret of their success? Knowing what your mailman knows.

Back in the late 1990s, congressional Republicans fought bitterly with the Clinton White House over Medicare. As part of the budget negotiations of 1997, they hatched a compromise: a bipartisan commission would be established to recommend reforms. It was inevitable that the committee, riddled with partisan appointments, would fail to get the supermajority vote required to make recommendations to Congress. But if the commission technically failed, the majority did agree on the first step toward a more sensible program: premium support.

To understand premium support and the basic thrust of the commission's recommendations, we again need to step back four decades. Before Medicare and Medicaid, in 1959, members of Congress established a government program that served a more immediate interest: their own. The Federal Employee Health Benefits Program was designed not simply for congressmen and their families, but for all interested federal employees. Today, it covers nine million, roughly 85 percent of the total federal workforce.

There are numerous similarities between Medicare and the FEHBP, as Harry Cain, a former vice president of BlueCross BlueShield, points out:

> Medicare and the FEHBP are alike in several ways. Both began in the 1960s, both provide relatively generous benefits (although the FEHBP's are more generous), and both cover very large populations (although Medicare's is four times larger). Both prohibit medical underwriting, age rating, and waiting periods for preexisting conditions. No one eligible to join either program can be excluded. As federally legislated programs, both also override the states' relevant laws. Thus, they both are reasonably uniform in their operation across the country. Both are providing what they were set up to provide, although they were set up very differently.[25]

But there are also enormous differences. Unlike Medicare, the program is not run by Washington but is rather a composite of private plans. On this account, the contrast between Medicare and the FEHBP could not be greater. Consider: for much of the last decade, Washington has debated how to add a prescription drug benefit to Medicare—and now, how to implement it—but the FEHBP already covers prescription drugs.

The reason why Medicare has lacked a drug benefit is simple. In 1965, Wilbur Mills didn't think much about outpatient prescriptions because pharmaceuticals were a small part of health care. That wasn't a reflection on Mills' ambition so much as on the state of medicine then; in fact, he modeled Medicare after the standard Blue Cross policies of his time. Today, it seems almost inconceivable not to have prescription drug coverage in a Blue Cross plan or any other private plan—thus the debates in Washington. But Medicare has remained structurally frozen in time. In contrast, the FEHBP has evolved since its creation; none of the participating health insurance policies lacks a drug benefit.

Robert Moffit explains that the FEHBP is based on three simple principles.

Choice. Federal workers can choose from a wide variety of plans. Options include HMOs, PPOs (preferred provider organizations), and fee-for-service policies. Consumer-driven health insurance is now in the mix. There is even a faith-based plan on the model of a health savings account. Obviously, the availability of plans depends on where a person lives. But no federal employee has fewer than a dozen options, even those living in rural areas.

Competition. With so much choice, insurance plans are directly competing for consumer dollars. In all, there are over 240 plans. Federal employees can pick and choose what best meets their needs. There is also information available to guide the choices—including a publication detailing the differences among the plans.

Light Regulation. The federal government doesn't specify a comprehensive list of standard benefits. Just as important, the program is free of state regulations, like mandated benefits and premium taxes.

Employees covered by the FEHBP are thus given a menu of options from a host of participating companies that offer plans meeting minimal requirements. In terms of payment, the federal government offers premium support—that is, a percentage of the premium is picked up by Washington, depending on the expense of the plan.[26] In other words, the federal government's role in the FEHBP is to pay the bills; under Medicare, Washington is the designer of benefits.

There are two central questions to ask with regard to Medicare reform: Does the FEHBP really work? Is it relevant to Medicare?

Yes, it works.

Measuring the success of a health plan is complex. But by several measures, the FEHBP works.

First, it's popular among recipients. A full 85 percent of federal employees are signed up—a high participation rate. Are they satisfied? In a 2003 survey, 79 percent of non-HMO enrollees and 63 percent of HMO enrollees rated their plans at 8 or higher on a scale of 10.[27]

That result is hardly surprising. After all, the FEHBP allows federal employees to vote with their feet. Every year, there is an "open season" when employees pick their plan for the following year. An employee who is dissatisfied with his HMO or dislikes some aspect of a PPO can simply switch plans. (Every year, about 5 percent do.) This puts tremendous pressure on health plans to be competitive and innovative. Not surprisingly, most are. Ideas like disease management and pharmacy benefit management (PBM)—ideas that are debated as reform ideas for Medicare—have been part and parcel of some FEHBP plans for years. And the diversity of choices is great. For instance, the vast majority of employers in America don't offer consumer-driven plans. In 2006, there were nineteen such plans in the FEHBP.

If employees enjoy the options, the federal government has plenty of reason to celebrate as well. The FEHBP is pretty cost-effective. Whereas private companies—even big corporations—fret about the extraordinary rise in health expenditures in recent years, the FEHBP has been excellent at keeping spending in check. Over a two-decade period, private insurance spending has soared 9.1 percent annually. The FEHBP costs, in contrast, have risen 6.5 percent annually. Only Medicare has been better at holding the line on spending. But remember two things about Medicare: First, administrators cheat, since they hold the line on spending partly by price fixing. Indeed, Medicare is one of the most elaborate price-control schemes in history, with Washington setting the price on 7,000 medical procedures offered by 800,000 physicians and other professionals. Second, Medicare benefits to date have not covered outpatient prescription drugs. To compare the FEHBP to Medicare in a meaningful way, we should factor out pharmaceuticals.[28] When we do, the FEHBP bests Medicare at controlling costs. As Harry Cain remarks, "The FEHBP has out-performed Medicare every which way—in containment of costs, both to consumers and to the government, in benefits ... inno-vation and modernization, and in consumer satisfaction."[29]

Percent of Annual Spending Growth per Capita
for Major Health Insurers, 1983–2002[30]

Medicare	6.7
FEHBP	6.5
FEHBP without drugs	5.8
Private Insurance	9.1
Medicaid	7.1
GDP	4.9

Source: Joint Economic Committee

Yes, it's relevant.

The FEHBP may be a decent way to insure federal employees, but would such an approach actually improve Medicare? Certainly there is the potential to address some of the most basic problems with Medicare. The FEHBP holds costs down—without price control. It offers choice and competition, and it includes drug coverage.

Looking to the FEHBP as a potential model for Medicare is not an obscure idea, applauded in academic circles but rarely considered outside the ivory towers. As we noted before, Senator John Breaux and Congressman Bill Thomas headed the National Bipartisan Commission on the Future of Medicare. They considered various ideas for reforming Medicare, eventually settling on a proposal that was modeled after the FEHBP.

The Breaux-Thomas proposal was built on three ideas:

1. There is no point in having a Medicare Part A and Part B; there should simply be one Medicare.
2. The best way to address Medicare's shortcomings is to drop the present model and instead offer competing private plans.
3. The federal government should offer premium support, with more subsidies for lower-income seniors than for those with higher incomes.

A majority on the commission voted in favor of the Breaux-Thomas proposal; but that wasn't enough to recommend changes to Congress, since the mandate of the commission had required a supermajority. The following year, Senator Breaux and Senator Bill Frist proposed a more saleable version of the commission's proposal. Again, the approach was to replace Medicare with several competing plans; again, they envisioned premium support. This time, however, they were generous and politically sensitive. Unfortunately, the plan was lost in the 2003 drive for a prescription drug benefit. Whereas a bipartisan coalition had sought to overhaul Medicare in the late 1990s, a Republican majority succeeded in expanding it with no overhaul in 2003.

Breaux-Thomas is something of a breakthrough, though, and a good place to start the discussion on Medicare reform. For one thing, their compromise managed to achieve some level of bipartisan agreement. Just as important, the push was to reform Medicare, not simply to grow it. In fact, the commission carefully scored the recommendations, suggesting that the Breaux-Thomas approach would shave between 1.0 and 1.5 percent a year from the program's growth.

Can we use the principles of Breaux-Thomas to reform Medicare?

How to Reform Medicare

Let's pick up where the National Bipartisan Commission on the Future of Medicare left off. We can reform Medicare by bringing in choice and competition. Here's how:

1. *Raise the qualifying age.* People live longer and healthier than ever before. Yet Washington makes the same requirement of beneficiaries—that they have turned 65—as Medicare did in 1965. Shouldn't we update our definition of a senior? In 1983, Congress did exactly that with another entitlement, Social Security. In 2003, the retirement age began moving up from 65 and eventually will hit 67. (The change, however, is to be phased in over 24 years.) If Social Security can update its definition of a senior, why doesn't Medicare? Such a modest change would help with solvency. Indeed, targeting 70 would seem reasonable.

2. *Simplify the insurance.* Medicare is divided into several plans. Mills' original legislation created Part A (for hospitals) and Part B (for outpatient services), in part reflecting the debate at the time. In the 1990s, Part C was added, allowing managed care. Now there is a prescription drug benefit, Part D. Finally, most Medicare beneficiaries have supplementary insurance and pay out of pocket. Such a division is unnatural. Under Part D, for example, Medicare beneficiaries will be the only group in America buying health insurance just for prescription drugs (a bit like buying home insurance only for the basement). Such an approach isn't just convoluted, it's redundant. The National Center for Policy Analysis hired an actuary, Mark Litgow, to analyze present spending on prescription drugs. He concluded that it would have been possible for Congress to add a prescription drug benefit for Medicare *without* spending more public money, as long as seniors could have combined their Medigap and out-of-pocket expenditures into one plan.

3. *Allow choice.* Just as with the FEHBP, Medicare should allow beneficiaries to choose among competing private plans. Rather than take a heavy regulatory approach as was done with Medicare + Choice (Part C), Washington should set minimal requirements and allow participation from different types of plans. Under Breaux-Thomas, seniors would have full premium support for insurance that covered the benefits of Parts A and B. Seniors who want more would then pay more.

4. *Add choices.* With the Medicare Modernization Act of 2003, all Americans can now purchase health savings accounts—except elderly Americans. But many seniors would appreciate HSAs, for the same reasons that younger people do: HSAs empower people with health dollars, giving them the options and flexibility they want. As well, if seniors are content with their present insurance (because, for example, they continue to work), it makes sense to allow them to opt out of Medicare.

5. *Support the elderly intelligently.* Presently, Medicare treats elderly Americans more or less equally.[31] In the new prescription drug benefit, a Walton or a Vanderbilt has access to the same coverage under Part D that an Arkansan or New Yorker with a less august name (and bank account) would have.[32] If elderly

Americans want more benefits—comprehensive drug coverage, for example—then they should pay more for the plan. Premium support is a reasonable way of helping Medicare recipients. Furthermore, the support should adjust for incomes and assets.

6. *Support the elderly intelligently, continued.* The FEHBP is insensitive to a recipient's health. This makes sense for a plan that covers a group of citizens who, collectively, are relatively healthy: federal employees. But Medicare insures the elderly, and there can be wide variation in the health status of recipients. Obviously, this poses a problem in a program that allows individuals the option of switching policies regularly. A reformed Medicare will need to adjust for risk, paying more for those who are sicker.

7. *Regulate lightly.* One of the most important aspects of the FEHBP is that regulations are light. But Medicare is the opposite, filled with numerous rules and regulations making it difficult for private companies to enter; witness the debacle of Medicare + Choice. To allow the private plans to participate and flourish with little interference from Washington, Medicare should be spun off from the Centers for Medicare and Medicaid Services, governed by a separate agency.

Ultimately, Medicare needs to offer a variety of options for seniors—not simply to help address the insolvency issue, but to deliver better care for America's elderly. With proper risk-adjusting, Medicare would become (in John Goodman's phrase) a "market for sick people." Insurance companies would specialize and then advertise to recruit seniors. So, for example, after a Florida retiree suffers a heart attack, plans will compete for his Medicare dollars, offering specialized cardiac care.

These seven steps will not solve all of Medicare's troubles in one swoop. But they do represent important progress on the most basic issues with the program. Consider how an FEHBP-style program might remedy the four I's of Medicare:

Insolvent. The Breaux-Thomas proposal offers some relief from Medicare's rising costs, aiming to trim spending by 1 to 1.5 percent a year. This is a welcome alternative to the present cost-containment strategy of price controls and limited benefits—but probably not enough in and of itself. If we pushed further than

Breaux-Thomas, as outlined above, the cost savings would almost surely be greater.

Inadequate. Given the chance to choose among plans, it's likely that many seniors would take their Medicare dollars and select more comprehensive insurance. In fact, many would probably opt for less first-dollar coverage, gaining instead provisions like catastrophic coverage. The point is that seniors would have a choice, finding the benefits that best met their needs.

Inefficient. An FEHBP-style program would help address the overinsurance issue. Many seniors would pick plans with deductibles and copays; others would go further, choosing HSA-style policies.

Inequitable. Geographic variation is a direct result of Medicare's overinsurance of recipients. Montana residents aren't worrying about the higher incidence of back surgery in their state than in, say, New York, because they aren't affected by the costs of the overservicing. Move decisions closer to recipients, and important questions will be asked.

SLOWLY BUT SURELY, WASHINGTON IS beginning to address its immediate fiscal woes with a bipartisan call for greater discipline. Getting the federal budget—and thus the federal deficit—under control is a worthy goal. But it is unrealistic in the long term unless Washington is willing to do something about Medicare.

In a way, Medicare reform was debated more meaningfully a decade ago, when Republicans and Democrats acknowledged its long-term problems. The introduction of a prescription drug benefit confused and sidetracked discussion of Medicare reform. The president began by asking for Medicare reform and a drug benefit, but ended up with just a drug benefit. The result was to exacerbate what was already a problem in American health care: the economics of prescription drugs.

EIGHT

Our Drug Problem

"Merck's $27 Billion Heart Attack: Lawyers are circling. Wall Street is howling. Can the proud drug giant survive the Vioxx mess?"
—*Fortune* magazine cover, November 1, 2004

IT'S DIFFICULT NOT TO MARVEL at the quick demise of Vioxx. The drug's release in 1999 was an absolute success: Vioxx quickly became a blockbuster with over 100 million prescriptions, 20 million users and $2.5 billion in annual sales.[1] Vioxx and its sister drugs belonged to a novel class of analgesics, the COX-2 inhibitors—medications that alleviate pain for millions of Americans without the gastric complications of NSAIDs. Vioxx represented everything *right* about American pharmaceuticals. Millions of baby boomers happily spent a few dollars per pill and forgot the way a medicine cabinet looked without a bottle or two of Vioxx in it.

Until, one day, it all exploded with a bombshell announcement: Merck would withdraw Vioxx from the market. Suddenly, Vioxx represented everything *wrong* with American pharmaceuticals, and millions wondered how it ever got into their medicine cabinets. Merck's share price dropped by one-third in a single day.

While the FDA would eventually allow Merck's former wunderkind back on the market, the damage was great. Merck lost more than share price: its CEO was pushed out and the company now seems ripe for a takeover. The collateral damage hit the FDA, with new cries for reform of the agency.[2]

Merck's heart attack seemed to confirm the worst suspicions of the American public: pharmaceuticals like Vioxx are too expensive and, to boot, not necessarily safe. Not surprisingly, there is now a populist, bipartisan push to regulate the drug industry more carefully—and some are going further, demanding that even prices be regulated in the form of reimportation.

If a populist movement capitalizes on American discontent, there is good reason. Americans have never been more ambivalent about their medications: Americans like state-of-the-art drugs, but not the pharmaceutical companies that make them; Americans celebrate the success of pharmaceutical innovation, but bemoan the high cost of funding it.

As with so much of American health care, the problems that politicians are eager to discuss have little to do with the underlying issues in pharmaceutical policy. First and foremost, there are the same problems that permeate the rest of American health care, like employer-sponsored health insurance or Medicaid. For historic reasons, the financing and regulation of prescription drugs are deeply colored by third-party payership and paternalism. Three central issues are:

- Americans don't pay directly for the drugs they consume, leading to high costs but not necessarily always better health.
- The FDA is overly rigorous in its demands, driving up the cost of drug development.
- Limited follow-up is done on drugs after approval, meaning that trial lawyers (not scientists) have the final say on drug withdrawals.

This ties in with the problems of American health care—paternalism and government overregulation. As we outline in this chapter, choice and competition are the key to the solution.

Importing a Bad Idea

Has yellow ever looked so beautiful as it did when, in July 2005, Lance Armstrong rode victoriously on the Champs-Elysees, wearing the Tour de France's bright yellow jersey, reserved for champions? And what a champion! Armstrong had cycled his way to seven straight triumphs in the grueling 2,000-mile race—more wins than anyone in the history of cycling. But here's the irony: at the time Armstrong was flattening his opponents, a bipartisan coalition was promoting an idea that would flatten the industry that made it all possible. This juxtaposition speaks volumes about criticisms of the pharmaceutical industry.

Lance Armstrong is a cancer survivor, having prevailed over advanced testicular cancer, with twelve tumors in his lungs and two in his brain. His story of illness and recovery is now well known. But here's a detail that is too often glossed over: just thirty years ago, testicular cancer was a death sentence. Twenty years ago, treatment helped extend life expectancy but it was harsh, often lasting two years. Today, 96 percent of Americans survive the illness, just as Mr. Armstrong did, and the biggest improvement in care has been better drugs. Chemotherapy today takes under three months and is highly effective.

The pharmaceutical revolution has played a critical role in the awesome progress of medicine in the past sixty years. Think of antibiotics that stop infection; beta-blockers that reduce heart attack mortality by a third; antihypertensives that prevent heart attacks in the first place; and the chemo agents that helped Lance Armstrong. "I owe my life to cancer research," he has said.[3]

Yet, looking across the Western world, it would seem as if the pharmaceutical industry were engaged in frivolous activity rather than lifesaving work. In the 1980s, people spoke of a war on drugs. Today, there's a war on drug companies. The contradictions are palpable: if drugs have never done more, Americans have never been more ambivalent about the industry that makes them. Half of American adults have an unfavorable opinion of drug companies[4]—an amazing statistic considering that 44 percent of Americans take at least one prescription drug. While there are significant issues in pharmaceutical policy—in the way the United States regulates and pays for its drugs—the critics have cemented their opposition into a single disastrous idea: drug reimportation.

The idea sounds neat enough. In countries like Canada, prescription drugs are price-controlled. Reimportation means bringing drugs made by large pharmaceutical companies—many of them American—across the border from countries like our northern neighbor. The result, we are told, would be American innovation and American products at Canadian prices.

For a growing list of politicians, academics, and activists, reimportation is an idea whose time has come. Consider, for example, the angry comments of Congressman Dan Burton, a conservative Republican from Indiana: "It's about money, the money that the pharmaceutical companies are making on the backs of the American people."[5] Burton is echoed by an impressive list of politicians at practically every level of government—from the mayor of Springfield, Massachusetts (pop. 150,000) to the governor of Illinois (pop. 12 million). Senator John McCain of Arizona, a Republican, favors reimportation, as does his Democratic colleague Max Baucus of Montana. Other champions include a former commissioner of the FDA, a former secretary of Health and Human Services, and a former surgeon general.

Reimportation is merely populism. If pharmaceutical products should be price-controlled, then Washington should act. But what is the point of (re)importing price controls? Indeed, there are various practical problems with the idea. For one thing, the Canadian pharmaceutical market serves a population one-tenth the size of the United States. There simply aren't enough drugs in Canadian drugstores for all of us here. Some proponents have thus suggested a "coercion" clause, forcing drug companies to sell to Canadian wholesalers, who would then sell to Americans.[6] But why the hassle if the ultimate goal is price controls?

Imported or otherwise, price controls don't make sense for pharmaceuticals, for the same reasons we dismiss them in other areas of the economy: they undermine profitability and thus choke off innovation. Reimportation advocates like to quote Canadian drug prices, but notice what they never mention: Canadian drug innovations. The country that produced insulin is now a backwater of drug development.

If Canada is known for its drug prices, the United States is known as the leader in cancer research. Consider the development of Avastin, a drug for treatment of bowel cancer. Unlike previous medications, Avastin aims at stopping angiogenesis, the process by which tumors cause blood vessels to grow in order to feed the cancerous cells—a novel approach in the fight against an ancient killer. There are, of course, many more American innovations. Partly because of the success of medical science, the number of Americans dying from cancer has dropped 1 percent a year since 1991, adjusting for age.[7] The best may be yet to come: in the next year, for example, two vaccines for cervical cancer will come to market.

This book is not an unqualified defense of pharmaceutical companies. I am certainly ambivalent about several industry practices: the drug dinners that mix education with advertising and wine, the highly paid drug reps, the skewed studies. I meet with drug reps periodically—I need the free samples to help my patients—and I find the process uncomfortable. We sit in my office and they lavish praise on me, laughing at my every joke. I'm not influenced by these meetings (and I don't even accept a cup of coffee from reps anymore), but I fear that too many of my colleagues are not of the same mind.

These misgivings aside, the issues around pharmaceuticals are far more complex than the reimportation crowd will acknowledge. The key is not to break the back of the pharmaceutical industry with price controls, but to create a market for medical progress.

Overinsured in America

For critics of pharmaceutical companies, the work of the Shark Fin Project represents everything that is wrong with the industry. AstraZeneca began the project in 1995 to prepare for the expiration of a patent in 2001. This was no ordinary patent: it protected the company's prized drug, the antiheartburn agent Prilosec, advertised as the Purple Pill. What AstraZeneca did—develop another Purple Pill and billions of dollars in new profit—exemplifies the lack of innovation that critics say is afflicting the industry. But absent from the analysis is a larger question: Why are consumers willing to buy expensive drugs if their benefit over less costly generics is not obvious?

Prilosec was one of the most commercially successful drugs in history. Originally, the Shark Fin group had hoped to replace

Prilosec with a more effective drug—but how could they improve on a medication that heals 90 percent of stomach ulcers in just two months? In the end, the group came up with a fudge—they created an isomer of Prilosec, meaning a mirror image of the original molecule, which they named Nexium.

As the *Wall Street Journal* reported, AstraZeneca commissioned four studies comparing Prilosec with Nexium.[8] The studies looked at stomach healing, but with Nexium at a double dose. Nevertheless, patients on Nexium did better in only two of the studies. In a direct head-to-head comparison at equivalent dosing, the difference in ulcer healing was a modest 3 percent (87 percent for Prilosec versus 90 percent for Nexium). If AstraZeneca's own data suggest limited difference between Prilosec and Nexium, would anyone really want the newer, more expensive drug? To encourage people to opt for Nexium, the company launched a half-billion-dollar advertising blitz and marketed the drug as the Purple Pill. The end result: another success story.

It is important to keep things in perspective. Nexium is just one drug. Damning the whole industry for a single product is like dismissing every computer company because the Commodore Amigo was a dud. On the other hand, the Nexium story is not a singular phenomenon, as Merrill Goozner explains in his critical account of the industry:

> The Prilosec-to-Nexium transition exemplified a common industry practice. Throughout the 1990s, the drug industry poured billions of research dollars into developing alternatives to drugs that were approaching the end of their patent terms. In most cases, the alternatives were little changed from the originals.[9]

Even a pharmaceutical vice president once told me over lunch, "When [reporter] Robert Pear calls me from the *New York Times* and asks me to explain how Nexium is a better drug, I can't."

Most critics regard this as simply a tale of corporate greed. But what the Prilosec-to-Nexium story primarily illustrates is the distorted medical marketplace. By comparison, consider that, at this moment, Sony and Microsoft are locked in a war over the multibillion-dollar gaming market. If Sony produced a new gaming system that offered nothing better than their old one at a higher cost, we know how the market would respond. American pharmaceuticals don't work like that because—as with the rest of American health care—people pay so little directly. Nexium may cost four dollars a pill, but most insured Americans pay only a modest copay, if anything. In fact, the out-of-pocket expenditures on prescription drugs have been dropping with time. In 1990, Americans directly paid 59 cents of every dollar spent on their pharmaceuticals; in 2000, they paid just 30 cents on the dollar. Couple this with the billions of dollars spent on direct-to-consumer advertising, and Americans have plenty of incentive to demand expensive drugs—and expensive consultations and expensive diagnostic testing—when cheaper alternatives exist.

This chapter opened with a discussion of the rise and fall of Vioxx. As a patented drug, Vioxx was expensive, especially compared with generic medications like naproxen. Below is a comparison of the annual costs of relief for arthritis pain. Vioxx exceeded naproxen in price by nearly ninefold. It is true that in specific situations, Vioxx *was* a better drug. But did Americans opt for the most appropriate drug for their own situation?

Annual Cost of Relief for Arthritis

Bextra 20 mg	$965
Vioxx 25 mg	$941
Celebrex 100 mg	$925
Ibuprofen 200 mg	$114
Naproxen 220 mg	$109

Source: National Center for Policy Analysis

In 2000, *Health Affairs* published a study on prescriptions of COX-2 inhibitors. Though now out of favor, COX-2s were considered a breakthrough, offering pain relief without the gastrointestinal side effects of NSAIDs. A group led by the University of Pennsylvania's Jalpa Doshi looked at nearly five thousand elderly Americans with osteoarthritis, considering their GI status and insurance coverage, and then following the drug they were prescribed for pain relief. The study concluded:

Aged Medicare beneficiaries with the most generous drug coverage and only moderate risk of a GI problem were actually more
likely to get a COX-2 (25 percent) than beneficiaries with no or
limited coverage but at substantial risk (20 percent). Among
those with the best coverage, GI risk had no independent effect
on who got the COX-2s. In other words, irrespective of the GI
risk, people with the most generous prescription plans in 2000
were more likely to use COX-2 inhibitors.

In sum, while drug coverage is clearly associated with
greater use of expensive COX-2 inhibitors, most of the increase
in use is among those least in need.[10]

Similar studies haven't been done on Nexium, but it wouldn't
seem farfetched to assume that Doshi's conclusions on COX-2s
in the Medicare population can be applied. Nexium isn't necessarily any better than Prilosec for most people—but generous
insurance benefits make that a moot point.

American health care will always be riddled with these sorts
of problems as long as people remain insulated from the consequences of their actions. With health savings accounts, by contrast, people spend their own health dollars, and so they begin
to ask questions. Does my heartburn really require a prescription? Can I get by with a generic or do I want a pill that costs four
dollars a day? Early data indicate that people with HSAs ask questions like these. Aetna, for example, offers employees a type of
consumer-directed health insurance. According to company data,
generic prescriptions grew by 13 percent, with a resulting 11 percent drop in total pharmacy charges.[11]

Pharmaceuticals should be one of the most transparent
aspects of American health care; because of FDA requirements
and the diligent work of scientists across the country, there are
a slew of studies for almost every drug, suggesting efficacy and
making comparisons with other drugs. For a person with high
cholesterol or acid reflux, the ability to comparison-shop is great.
What's missing today is an incentive to do so.

If payment for pharmaceuticals is skewed, what about their
regulation?

Ever Cautious at the FDA

Ask people at the Food and Drug Administration what they think of Dr. Henry Miller, and eyes roll. "He's just plain unhelpful," one official told me. Dr. Miller is a gadfly of sorts, one of the foremost critics of the FDA. To that end, he has churned out essays on the agency that have graced the pages of the *Wall Street Journal,* the *Los Angeles Times,* and the *New York Times.* To Dr. Miller, the FDA is a slow and wasteful organization. And he should know: he worked there for fifteen years. If we're serious about the future of American medicine, we need to consider his ideas.

Because the FDA's work falls largely off the public's radar, some may assume that its role is not very important. But the agency oversees the regulation of roughly 25 cents of every dollar spent by consumers. This includes the approval of all new pharmaceutical and biotech drugs and genetically modified foods. The FDA, in other words, has an impact on what's in your fridge and in your medicine cabinet.

The trouble is, the FDA may be the most risk-averse agency in America. Dr. Miller, who served as founding director of the FDA's Office of Biotechnology and now is a senior fellow at Stanford's Hoover Institution, tells a story of its bureaucratic malaise. He was in the group that reviewed the first biotech application: for manufacturing insulin through gene-splicing techniques. (Previously, insulin had come from the pancreases of cows and pigs by a slow and expensive process.) After four months of deliberation, and armed with reams of data on efficacy and safety, Dr. Miller's team was prepared to go ahead. But since drug approval time averaged two and a half years, his supervisor hedged, reasoning, "If anything goes wrong, think how bad it will look that we approved the drug so quickly."[12] Dr. Miller waited until his supervisor went on vacation and then got approval from his supervisor's boss. In Miller's view, the process is still too slow nearly a quarter century after the insulin approval in 1982.

At the same time, many critics argue the other side of the issue, claiming that the FDA is simply too loose in its requirements, thereby not properly protecting America's drug supply. Post-Vioxx, the big push is to enlarge the FDA. The *Lancet* warned

that "patients' lives will continue to be endangered" without better regulation.

It seems that everyone dislikes the agency. Dr. Miller quotes
a former FDA commissioner, Frank Young, in characterizing the
agency as "a slow-moving target that bleeds profusely when hit."
But is it too over-reaching or too small?

The temptation with regulation is to think only in terms of
safety. If we check, say, two thousand patients for side effects, is
it possible that the drug will come to market and then harm some
patients? Maybe we should test the drug on more people: why
not three or four thousand? By being more rigorous, we could
prevent future suffering of patients.

That's the thinking behind increasingly rigorous standards
for approval at the FDA. In the mid-1980s, the average drug trial
involved 1,300 patients; today, the typical drug is tested on 4,300
people. The FDA is even stricter with applications for primary-
care drugs. Since a new drug for high blood pressure is unlikely
to offer a significant breakthrough in treatment, the FDA demands
more evidence of safety. Advanced clinical trials for antihypertensives involve 10,000 patients or more. A recent trial for a blood
thinner involved some 30,000 people.[13]

But there is a flip-side to this approach: by dwelling so heavily on safety, the FDA prevents drugs from coming to market. Sure,
many people must be tested to assure safety for patients in the
future, but what about today's patients who might benefit from
a drug? Back in 1988, the FDA approved misoprostol, using data
suggesting that the drug might save between 8,000 and 15,000
lives a year.[14] Certainly that's an amazing development—a new
drug that will save thousands of lives. But how many people died
because of the time it took to bring the drug to market?[15]

A balancing act is necessary between ensuring that patients
are safe and ensuring a market for medical progress. But the
dynamics of the FDA are skewed, as a former FDA commissioner,
Alexander Schmidt, has observed:

> In all our FDA history, we are unable to find a single instance
> where a Congressional committee investigated the failure of
> FDA to approve a new drug. But the times when hearings have
> been held to criticize our approval of a new drug have been so

frequent that we have not been able to count them. The message to FDA staff could not be clearer.[16]

The handling and eventual withdrawal of Rezulin is a case in point. Everyone can agree that Rezulin did a good job of controlling the blood sugar of patients with diabetes, particularly those who didn't respond well to insulin. Rezulin had a serious problem, however. It caused liver toxicity in some patients. Fortunately, this could be predicted with a simple blood test.

So the FDA issued multiple warnings to doctors, advising them to check liver-function tests and not to prescribe the drug to certain high-risk patients. Doctors continued to prescribe it anyway. At one point, as the story goes, a senior administrator at the FDA threw up his hands and said, "We can't trust doctors anymore to do the right thing." A different interpretation would be that doctors were doing the right thing in their estimation— they just had a different risk/benefit analysis than the FDA.

Eventually, the FDA held hearings on Rezulin. Despite pleas from countless patients, Warner-Lambert (now Pfizer) was pressured to withdraw the drug and it did so. But if the Rezulin controversy is largely forgotten outside the FDA, it proved to be a tipping point of sorts within the agency, resulting in greater caution. Consider some recent decisions:

• The original aim of the FDA was to act as an informed filter for the public. Information would be submitted and analyzed, and then the FDA would release its conclusions. The agency is now doing the opposite. For example, the FDA comments on "emerging risks"—releasing data that they've seen and are concerned about, but can't yet draw conclusions from.

• Despite the positive recommendation of an expert panel on silicone implants, the FDA balked at approval (perhaps because of political pressure from feminists). Again, it seems to be a case of good public relations winning out over good patient protection. A similar positive recommendation on Plan B, an emergency contraceptive, failed to result in approval (pressure, this time, being mounted by social conservatives).

• The FDA ordered Iressa, a cancer medication, off the market with a requirement of further clinical testing. The chemo agent shows a good result (10 percent) for a previously deadly cancer. Still, bureaucrats are unhappy that the drug doesn't show more robust results as compared with an off-label use of another pharmaceutical. Months before, the FDA had used similar logic in a decision not to fast-track Marquibo, also an anticancer agent.

• For two years, the FDA procrastinated on approving Erbitux, arguing that it lacked adequate data for this oncology drug. Eventually, the FDA gave the green light—acting, incidentally, on the same data set that it previously deemed inadequate.

ImClone, the maker of Erbitux, has been in the news because the household maven Martha Stewart is alleged to have sold company shares using insider information, thereby saving herself some $50,000. But thousands of patients with advanced colon cancer didn't have the chance to benefit from this effective drug while the FDA delayed its approval. Which is the real scandal? Erbitux was a clear example of the FDA's sloth. But there is a subtler issue: the cancer-drug pipeline is hardly robust. Vanderbilt University researchers recently concluded that during 1999–2004 there was a 68 percent reduction in new drug approvals from the preceding five-year period. The bigger pharmaceutical picture isn't much brighter. Despite billions in new research spending, the number of drug approvals has barely budged annually since the 1970s.

Part of the problem is the FDA's excessive regulations. Since 1964, the total time required for drug development, from synthesis of the molecule to marketing approval, has more than doubled, now topping fifteen years. It's not just the incredible delay that's problematic: according to the Tufts Center for the Study of Drug Development, pharmaceutical companies spend almost $900 million to bring a drug to market. Thirty years ago, the cost was a small fraction, $138 million (adjusted for inflation). The bureaucratic hurdles, in other words, have been set too high. FDA caution is undermining our ability to make new drugs and save lives.

The FDA's bureaucratic malaise is a major problem. How to solve it?

Faster Drug Approvals

Changing the FDA is no simple task—and it's no surprise that several presidencies have come and gone without fundamental change. But it's important to remember why the FDA needs to change. Sandy Britt illustrates the point well. A 46-year-old resident of Alameda, California, Ms. Britt was diagnosed with a stage IV lung cancer—meaning that the cancer cells had spread throughout her body. "The first doctor gave me a death sentence," she told the *Wall Street Journal*. "She wasn't even going to treat me."[17] Fortunately, Ms. Britt found a more aggressive physician. After running some genetic tests, he concluded that she might respond to a new pharmaceutical. "I've had an amazing response to it. They predicted I'd be dead now. Instead, I just got back from three weeks in Italy." Ms. Britt responded to Iressa—but it's no longer available to cancer patients because of bureaucratic obstruction. Patients like Sandy Britt deserve better.

Here are some steps for reforming the FDA.

1. *Apply some pressure.* Sunshine and common sense are a partial antidote to regulatory overkill. Former FDA commissioner Alexander Schmidt hit the nail on the head—congressional pressure now takes the form of demands for greater safety. It would be refreshing instead to ask hard questions of FDA officials. Why is Iressa off the market? Why is the drug pipeline not more robust? A few hearings on these topics would be worthwhile and could tap more than industry representatives worrying about regulatory hurdles. A diverse coalition of groups has a vested interest in such matters: AIDS activists, scientists, patient advocacy groups.

2. *Take the FDA leadership seriously.* There are long periods of time when the FDA is, effectively, without leadership—that is, the organization is between "permanent" commissioners and is run by an acting commissioner. President George W. Bush's first term would be a case in point. It's true that the president did choose a capable and intelligent physician, Dr. Mark McClellan, to run the agency—and then promptly promoted him out of the position. During the first four years of President Bush's administration, the FDA had a permanent commissioner for just fifteen

months. (The choice of Lester Crawford—a career bureaucrat with the FDA—to lead the organization for the second term hardly seemed inspired.)

3. *Reduce the overlap with other agencies.* The FDA shouldn't be reinventing the wheel. Yet it does: drugs that are approved in Europe are subjected to a battery of new tests before being considered for the American market. Given that the European Medicines Agency's drug approval times are just as long as the FDA's, it isn't clear that a drug really requires a slew of new tests. Reciprocity would save time and money.

4. *Change the incentives at the FDA.* If caution is the central dynamic of the FDA's bureaucracy, insensitivity to complaint is its approach to customer service. There is limited ability for a company or patient group to appeal decisions. Some, including Henry Miller, champion a simple idea: create an ombudsman to act in the public interest. This office, independent of the commissioner, would have the ability to criticize and take action against FDA employees found to be responsible for flawed decisions that constitute severe, avoidable errors. An ombudsman's office wouldn't be a panacea, but it could help counter the bureaucratic malaise.

These steps are all reasonable and easily done. But if we're really serious about shortening drug approval times, we must change the process itself.

At present, drug companies work through various stages as they take a drug to market. First, there is the *discovery phase,* when a company attempts to find an interesting chemical. If the results are suggestive of a promising compound, the company begins *pre-clinical testing*—that is, animal testing. After this, the company must apply to the FDA to go to the next step: the *clinical trials.* If the FDA gives the green light, the compound is introduced to humans, initially with a small group of healthy volunteers (Phase I) and then with larger (Phase II) and even larger (Phase III) groups including people who are ill, to study efficacy, side effects, and adverse reactions. When all the testing is done, the FDA is sent a *New Drug Application*—hundreds of thousands of pages of clinical data describing the response people had to the drug. The application also includes everything from the packaging of the drug, to its manufacturing, to the proposed labeling.

Now the ball is in the FDA's court. With the help of statisticians, pharmacologists, physicians, lawyers, and others, the FDA considers whether or not to approve the drug. The final stage of consideration is rarely a simple yes or no; the FDA often requires further data or asks for application revisions.

The last step is a bottleneck, taking months, sometimes years. Much of this holdup, however, has nothing to do with difficult decisions being considered by esteemed members of the scientific community. Rather, with so much data to analyze and only so many staff, the FDA takes time to work through a New Drug Application.

With an eye on this bottleneck, Congress passed the Prescription Drug User Fee Act of 1992. The idea was simple: introduce user fees, allowing the FDA to hire more staff. With more resources, approval times should decrease. As Daniel Carpenter, a Harvard professor, and his co-authors note in a *Health Affairs* study, approval times have in fact dropped for this final stage.

But does all the number crunching and statistical work actually have to be done in-house? If final approval rests with the FDA, isn't there room to contract out some of the work? President George H. W. Bush's administration asked this question in the late 1980s. The FDA took up the challenge, embarking upon a two-year pilot program. New Drug Applications were reviewed at the FDA, but also evaluated by the Mitre Corporation, a nonprofit company. For all five applications, the FDA analysts reached the same conclusion as their nongovernment peers. Significantly, though, the Mitre Corporation's reviews cost a fraction of the FDA's and were completed in an amazingly short two to four months. But these results are not surprising; the FDA is notorious for its sluggishness.

This approach may seem novel for drug approval, but many nonprofits are in the business of reviewing the safety of other kinds of products. Think of the work done by Consumer Union (publishers of *Consumer Reports*) and Underwriters Laboratories.

To clear up the FDA's biggest bottleneck without significantly reconsidering safety and efficacy requirements, the agency should allow companies the option of an external review, financed by user fees. Such a move would be cost-neutral to the FDA—

but, judging from the pilot program, it would lead to faster reviews. The FDA is presently a certifier of products. With external contracting, the FDA would increasingly become a certifier of certifiers—reviewing the reviewers, rather than exercising day-to-day oversight of drug approvals. Some, such as Henry Miller, have suggested that the drug approval process become a competitive market of nongovernment reviewers analyzing the data, ultimately making recommendations to the FDA. Reviewers would be able to charge a user fee. Organizations that could offer faster reviews at lower fees would clearly attract the business of pharmaceutical companies seeking approval for their products.

It's not difficult to foresee the objections of industry critics like Public Citizen. In the eyes of these so-called consumer advocates, a marketplace for drug reviews would be akin to a market for shoddy standards. But is this argument actually borne out in the wider marketplace? Let's consider the Underwriters Laboratories, which has certified most things electric in your home. (If you're skeptical, look for the distinctive UL logo on, say, your desk lamp; the company claims that the average household will have 125 of these logos.) Underwriters Laboratories charges fees to certify products. But far from undermining standards, the organization recognizes that its certification is only as good as its reputation. To address any concerns about conflict of interest, its board includes insurance company executives, former public servants, and consumer advocates. If such an approach is good enough to keep you from being electrocuted, why couldn't it keep you from being poisoned?

Safer Drugs

Call it the post-Vioxx conventional wisdom: the belief that approval standards must be toughened up to ensure that America's drugs are safe. Indeed, many demand that the FDA require more clinical trials on greater numbers of participants, with the logic that the system has failed spectacularly so we should embrace the system more zealously. Here's the FDA's dirty little secret: clinical trials involve a relatively homogeneous group of healthy individuals who collectively are totally unrepresentative of the people who actually take pharmaceuticals. The FDA doesn't need to raise the bar higher, it needs to rethink drug safety.

It's not just the choice of participants for clinical trials that is problematic for screening potential adverse effects. Statistically speaking, clinical trials involve few people; if a drug effect has a very low prevalence rate, it's unlikely to be noticed in a clinical trial involving a few thousand. That's why even relatively large clinical trials—such as those involving tens of thousands of people—are ultimately unable to reveal the adverse events that precipitate drug withdrawals. Only in real-world situations, with hundreds of thousands or even millions of users, can subtle problems be found. In other words, despite the extraordinary caution of the FDA, it's difficult to tell exactly how a drug affects people until it hits pharmacies. Bromfenac is a case in point. No problems had been discovered by the original clinical trials, involving 2,500 people. The analgesic was withdrawn after causing four deaths and necessitating eight liver transplants—but the medication was taken by 2.5 million people.[18]

The trouble here is that the whole regulation of pharmaceuticals is focused on approval. The FDA spends years demanding and poring over data, and then does almost no post-approval surveillance—thus, the Vioxx heart attack. Drug regulation in the United States is not unlike a university's tenure system: rigorous testing before approval, and then almost no follow-up. Perhaps that's a reasonable way to judge an academic, but is that really the ideal way to ensure that America's drugs are safe?

"Like death and taxes, drugs' side effects are inevitable," quips Henry Miller.[19] But in his view, the balance of accountability is wrong—overly weighed toward the approval side. He points out studies suggesting that in the United Kingdom, approximately 5 percent of hospital admissions are in some way due to an adverse effect of a medicine; and between 5 and 10 percent of hospitalized patients are estimated to suffer an adverse drug experience.

Increasing the number of participants in clinical trials will not remedy this problem, but only add to the overall cost of drug development. "The approval process for a new drug—the part of the drug development process that involves testing new medicines in people—can already take as long as ten years and costs as much as $466 million," remarks Dr. Scott Gottlieb, now the deputy commissioner of the FDA. "Some cardiovascular drugs are tested in clinical trials that enroll 10,000 patients or more at an average cost of $20,000 per patient."[20]

Instead of longer clinical trials, what's needed is post-approval surveillance, based on two types of information: data from the point of care (doctors who prescribe) and practical clinical data culled from real-world settings (drug companies, insurance companies, and Medicare). But today, neither source of information is particularly helpful.

Doctors are reluctant to take the time to fill out lengthy drug safety reports. Some have estimated that under 1 percent of adverse events are reported by doctors. Indeed, the FDA has so little confidence in safety information coming from physicians' offices that they have a full-time staff whose job it is to read medical journals for letters about drug reactions, figuring that doctors are actually more likely to write to a journal than to the FDA. Meanwhile, drug companies seem to do the opposite, flooding the FDA with any and every possible adverse reaction, burying significant events in a graveyard of data.[21] This over-reporting creates distracting noise. On top of this, the FDA largely doesn't monitor post-approval side effects anyway.

So who has the ultimate say in drug withdrawals? Trial lawyers. It is the threat of litigation that causes drug companies to consider carefully whether or not a drug ought to stay on the market. When the FDA warned about the possible liver effects of Rezulin, the agency didn't order a withdrawal. It didn't have to— the manufacturer pulled the drug from the nation's pharmacies, fearing litigation. And the Vioxx withdrawal wasn't motivated so much by a profound concern over company data as by fear of the trial lawyers. (Merck's gambit turned out to be a dud, as some 36,000 lawsuits were launched.)

Dr. Gottlieb finds a potential solution in information technology. Electronic medical records, for example, could be used to follow patients' reactions to new drugs:

> If a new drug is launched that has a certain rare toxicity to the
> liver, a real-time surveillance network might eventually be able

to detect subtle elevations in the liver enzyme tests of patients who were started on the drug and also happened to have blood work done around the same time. If enough of these signals were detected, it might alert the FDA that there is a potential liver toxicity and allow the agency to intervene before real harm is done to any patients.[22]

Electronic medical records are not the standard in many hospitals and clinics, but they are used in enough hospitals and clinics to provide a substantial information base. As well, there are good tools already available for accessing and manipulating data. The issue is not that the infrastructure doesn't exist, but rather that neither the FDA nor industry has invested in it.

Here, then, is a simple idea for improving drug safety without further enriching trial lawyers. The FDA, empowered by congressional action, should offer drug companies a deal: if they invest in post-approval monitoring—that is, pay for the information technology—and they provide all data to the FDA, they would in turn be protected from class-action lawsuits. The FDA could then meaningfully monitor adverse effects.

This would not be an unprecedented strategy; childhood immunization is handled in just this way. Vaccines carry small but defined risks. Vaccine makers are covered by a no-fault system—if a child becomes ill as a direct result of vaccination, his or her family is entitled to a set amount of money. Vaccine makers, however, cannot be sued by the family for more money.

Obviously, the situation is different with prescription drugs, since the risks are unknown. In the case of Vioxx, an expert advisory panel reviewed data from Kaiser and issued a warning about the cardiovascular risk. That's not a bad approach; but for too many drugs, the analysis isn't done or is done too late, depriving doctors and their patients of information on potential problems. Tort reform would provide a strong incentive for drug makers to work on post-approval monitoring. This would be a win-win for patients and pharmaceutical companies. The only losers would be trial lawyers.

The key is to maintain the innovation that drives pharmaceutical development. It's no accident that most drugs are developed in the United States, because European governments stifle innovation to a far greater degree than the FDA and the trial lawyers do.

Even so, critics of American health care routinely point to the European and Canadian systems as superior to our own. These systems may seem tempting because they are touted as lower in cost and higher in quality. In the next chapter, we consider these other systems in some detail.

NINE

The Hip That Changed History

IT'S NOT EVEN 9 A.M., but Dr. Brian Day bubbles with life. "It think we're finally moving forward," the Canadian surgeon tells me.[1] He laughs, shares stories of how he met Fidel Castro while volunteering in Cuba, and enthuses about the coming months. Dr. Day is the medical director and president of Cambie Surgical Centre, a private clinic in British Columbia. These days, he has much to celebrate—including Canada's shifting view of private medicine.

Despite our shared interests, Dr. Day and I have never met before this morning. Back in the mid-1990s, I wanted to write an article on his private clinic, but I couldn't find a newspaper interested in the pitch. Back then, Cambie was a small operation, focused on orthopedics.

Times have changed. Earlier this year, the *New York Times* interviewed Dr. Day. His clinic grows, covering a variety of surgical procedures, and there is talk of expansion to Calgary, Toronto, and Montreal. Dr. Day is now president-designate of the Canadian Medical Association. "I'm suddenly respectable," he jokes about the new title.

Life is not without complications. Dr. Day still faces a vote—and a potential challenge—in his presidential bid (the CMA's elections are only modestly less convoluted than a papal selection). The Ontario government warns of legal action if his clinic hangs a shingle in Canada's largest province. Yet Dr. Day is undaunted. He looks forward to representing the medical profession in the public eye and, if need be, his clinic in the courts of Ontario.

   The personal success of Brian Day reflects the remarkable change in Canadian attitudes toward private medicine. Not so long ago, Canadians wouldn't think of using the word "private" in the same sentence as "medicare"—their term for the publicly funded health-care system that so-called experts tout as the envy of the world. While Canadians reluctantly admitted there were some problems with the system, they argued that everything could be fixed with new public money. Talk of private health care was dismissed as "Americanization."

   Some in academia still speak in these terms. But most do not. Every week, one new private clinic opens in Canada. Dr. Day estimates that 50,000 British Columbians alone use some type of private health service every year, mainly diagnostics.

   Thus, in Dr. Day's success we see a remarkable phenomenon: after decades of acceptance, Canadians are reconsidering their health-care system. Whereas many Americans see government as a solution to the flaws of their own system, Canadians are now embracing a private alternative. Canadians have found that government-run health-care systems, far from being an elegant solution, are universally plagued with deep structural problems. In fact, whether we look to Canada or to Europe, we find that single-payer systems are fanciful temptations, like hoping that a new house will save a troubled marriage. As a result, politicians outside the United States are increasingly looking to individual choice and competition.

The Government Temptation

Government-run health care—what proponents now euphemistically call "single-payer"—is *not* poised to sweep the body politic and transform the nation. Indeed, it is an idea that exists in the shadows. When Oregon voted in 2002 on a ballot initiative promising Canadian-style health care, voters in the liberal bastion responded with uncharacteristic resolve, defeating Measure 23 by a 4 to 1 margin. "Like a sportswriter looking for synonyms to break up the monotony of saying one team beat another, Measure 23's fate—garnering barely 21% of the vote in favor—requires more action-oriented verbs such as shredded, pummeled, clobbered ... ," quipped Bill Virgin, a columnist for the *Seattle Post-Intelligencer.*[2]

National health care is not a dead idea. It is an enduring temptation, quietly capturing the imaginations of esteemed intellectuals and frustrated Americans. The *Los Angeles Times* muses wistfully that HillaryCare may not have been such a bad idea. Arnold Relman, former editor of the *New England Journal of Medicine,* describes the problems of American medicine in a 7,500-word essay for the *New Republic,* concluding that markets don't work. Matt Miller, a centrist in the Clinton administration's OMB, argues in *Fortune* that government-financed health care is a winning political idea—for Republicans. The National Coalition on Health Care, consisting of big businesses like General Electric and AT&T as well as union interests, announced support for a universal coverage scheme that would centralize key health decisions in a government committee. Legislatures in California, Ohio, and Vermont heatedly debated Canadian-style health care last year. In fifteen other states, bills have been introduced calling for the creation of a government-funded insurance scheme.

The problems with American health care are very real—the swelling ranks of the uninsured, the unease of the middle class, the frustration of everyone—and the desire to look elsewhere for answers seems reasonable. "My brother, a conservative small businessman, is saying maybe it's time for the government to take over health insurance," says Senator Susan Collins (R-Maine). "The one change I've noticed ... is that businesspeople for the first time are questioning whether private insurance can survive."[3] Dr. Marcia Angell, a former editor of the *New England Journal of Medicine,* says we need to recognize the "fatal flaw" in the system, which is that "we treat health care as a commodity," and consider a serious overhaul. "What we need is a national single-payer system that would eliminate unnecessary administrative costs, duplication and profits."[4]

True, there is limited enthusiasm on the part of federal politicians—especially in a Republican-dominated Congress—to take on a sweeping new initiative after the grand failure of the Clinton plan. True, too, that American journalists increasingly report the problems of single-payer systems like Canada's medicare. But

Americans would not dismiss the idea completely. It lives on because of its simplicity.

American health care is a vast and complicated system, involving trillions of dollars and hundreds of millions of individuals. It presents us with multiple challenges: How to deal with the uninsured? How to address workers' disappointment with rising copayments? What to do with cost escalation? The single-payer idea offers one simple answer to all these problems: government insurance. Those who promote the single-payer system present the idea as a magic bullet. Why fuss with the sticky economics of health care—adverse selection, supply-induced demand, information asymmetry, to name a few technical examples—when all you need is for the government to step forward?

But the solution is not so simple.

The Best Health Care in the World (Unless You're Sick)

Donna Longmoore and Christina Alcorn have similar problems, but they live in different worlds.[5] Both are diabetic. Both require insulin. Both grew tired of the seemingly endless injections and finger-prick blood tests. That's why these two women opted to get an insulin pump, a small device that fits comfortably on their belt and injects a steady stream of the lifesaving medicine into their bodies. It's cutting-edge technology and, not surprisingly, it carries a stiff price tag, roughly $5,000. But there the similarities end.

For Christina Alcorn, the pump was easy to obtain and was covered by her insurance company. For Donna Longmoore, it was a struggle, culminating in thousands of dollars of out-of-pocket expenses. In fact, most of the diabetics under Longmoore's plan don't have the pump, and many of the doctors don't even mention it to their patients. (Longmoore learned about the technology by chance when she was enrolled in an international diabetic study.)

The differences in these cases don't stop there. Alcorn sees an endocrinologist just a short drive away on a monthly basis. For Longmoore, access is more difficult. When her local endocrinologist would make her wait two to three hours, she finally decided to drive a bit farther to see her old specialist, who works two hours away. "At least I'm comfortable with him," she says. Despite her efforts, Longmoore will be lucky to see the specialist more than twice a year. Should she develop any diabetic complications, the wait to see another specialist—like an eye doctor or a kidney expert—may be weeks or, more likely, months. In contrast, Alcorn would wait days.

Is this difference in care a matter of wealth? Actually, both women are middle-class. Is Longmoore stuck in a restrictive HMO? It turns out that Alcorn is the one with the HMO coverage.

The difference ultimately is a matter of geography. Longmoore lives across the river from Alcorn—in Canada.

HEALTH-CARE SYSTEMS ARE COMPLICATED, and Canada's medicare is no exception. Whole books filled with inscrutable jargon attempt to explain its nuances. Health economists speak of Canada's system as being *a national health insurance with federal contributions, provincial administration and a for-profit but independent delivery of primary care within the context of a government-financed system.*

Yet Canadian medicare is relatively simple. Payment for most health services requires just one thing: a provincial plan number, given to every resident. Coverage, thus, is universal. For the most part, there are no copayments or deductibles, no laborious insurance forms, no difficult HMO bureaucrats. The plan covers everything that is "medically necessary," as the Canada Health Act declares. Most medical visits, diagnostic testing, and surgical procedures are covered.[6]

Shortly before Oregon's referendum on a single-payer health-care system, a man wrote to his local paper saying that under this system, "you just send your doctor's bill to the government and they pay it." But single-payer systems aren't quite so simple. It is true that patients don't need to fuss with insurance claims—doctors bill the government directly. But someone has to fund the labyrinth of services. In Canada, that someone is the provincial government.

Hospitals—all the hospitals—are thus funded by the government. Doctors work for the government, charging for services based on a billing schedule set by the state. But how much should hospitals receive for their budgets? How much should doctors get to bill? These questions are not easily answered; so it takes armies of government officials to administer Canadian medicare.

That the government must involve itself in determining the number of obstetrical beds in London, Ontario, seems like a small price to pay, or so argue many health economists on both sides of the 49th parallel. Consider the savings of a Canadian-style single-payer system: there is no duplication among plans; administrative costs are low; paperwork is kept to a minimum. As a result, some Canadian health-care experts still brag about their medicare. In late 2002, Roy Romanow (a former provincial premier) completed an exhaustive review of Canada's health-care system—a $10 million, eighteen-month federally commissioned effort. He concluded that the system is "efficient."

But efficiency can be measured by other criteria. For people waiting more than seven hours (on average) in the emergency rooms of Alberta's Capital Health Region, the system doesn't seem efficient. Nor for the 70 percent of Ontario cancer patients who wait for treatment longer than four weeks, the maximum wait acceptable to cancer specialists. Nor for the fifty Ontario patients who died waiting for a basic cardiac test in the late 1990s, according to a study published in the *Canadian Medical Association Journal* in 2002.

So Dr. Marcia Angell is right. Things *are* simple in Canada— unless you need care. It's a lesson I know too well.

My Waiting List Problem—and Ours

Health care touches everyone's life, and growing up in Canada I experienced firsthand the problems with a single-payer system. When I was finishing my medical training, my father complained of trouble walking. He had intense pain radiating down both his legs. At the time, he was in his sixties, a university professor who led an active life of teaching and research. He was particularly concerned when his grandchildren visited—he couldn't keep up.

He saw his family doctor, who wondered about a spinal problem. He was referred to a neurologist. The specialist would then work my father up and suggest treatment. As a Canadian citizen, my father needed nothing more than a health card for the consultation—and patience. The appointment was booked for three months later.

My father had increasing pain and decreasing mobility. At my graduation, he could barely walk a few steps. In the course of a few weeks, he had gone from an active life to the confines of his house. Searching out a second opinion, he went to an emergency room. "This isn't an emergency," he was told. "You just need to see a neurologist."

Herein lies the basic problem with Canadian health care: it's difficult to get things done. David Henderson, an economist who grew up in Canada, quips: "If you have a cold and are willing to wait in your family doctor's office for three hours, this is the best health-care system in the world." My father had more than a cold.

Seeing a neurologist would be just the first step. Surely, he would need an MRI. That would take months (typically, six). If the illness proved to be more serious, there would need to be a consultation with a neurosurgeon. The wait could be months more. If surgery was required, there could be a delay of further months.

Finally, my father decided to be proactive—he crossed the border. An MRI revealed spinal stenosis. Surgery was offered for the next day.

My father isn't the only one to have second thoughts about public health care. If angst is a reason to seek psychoanalysis, Canada's medicare seems to have transformed that nation into one ripe for a therapist's couch. A survey in 2000 involving 1,500 people suggested that a full eight out of ten Canadians consider their health-care system to be "in crisis."[7] Since then, polls consistently show health care as the top concern of voters. Medicare is the issue that dominates talk radio debates, peppers newspaper headlines, and colors election campaigns from coast to coast.

Buried deep in the fifth report from the Standing Senate Committee on Social Affairs, Science and Technology on the state of Canada's health-care system is a gentle reminder of why Canadians worry. The report details the struggle of a patient to get the care he needed. After being diagnosed with two herniated discs on April 19, 2001, the patient was promptly put on a waiting list for surgery. His procedure was classified as "elective but urgent"—a category that applies to most of the hospital's surgery cases. Eight months later, the patient testified before the committee. He had not had his surgery; it had not even been scheduled. Notes the report: "It appeared that the only way for the patient in question to move to the top of the list was for his condition to deteriorate. It was not enough for him to be in constant pain and unable to work."[8]

For those of us familiar with the Canadian health-care system, there's no difficulty giving examples of patients waiting too long for care. The head of family medicine at a large Montreal hospital told me that the system is so overwhelmed that emergency surgeries are often delayed. He relates the tale of an elderly man with a broken hip: while his orthopedic surgery was postponed for three days, he developed a blood clot and a potentially life-threatening pulmonary embolism.

These are anecdotes. But major studies, too, have exposed the same problems with the availability and timeliness of care:

- In an annual survey involving physicians across twelve different specialties, the Fraser Institute found that total wait times from the initial visit to the family doctor through to surgical therapy was 17.7 weeks. In every category, physicians thought wait times had exceeded "clinically reasonable" delays.[9]
- In the fall of 2000, the Canadian Association of Radiologists released a report saying that 63 percent of X-ray equipment was out of date, as was a majority of all diagnostic machinery in Canada. One-third of the radiological equipment in the city of Victoria, for example, was over two decades old.[10]
- In a major international study, the Heart and Stroke Foundation of Canada found that Canadian heart attack survivors have a dramatically lower quality of life than their U.S. counterparts. Among the findings: after twelve months, 31 percent of Canadians rated their health as better than in the month before the cardiac event; in the United States, 44 percent of survivors felt their health was better.[11]

There are many other studies pointing in the same direction.[12]

Why are Canadians forced to wait for the care they need? Patients face no user fees or deductibles for most health services, so health administrators have almost no ability to temper the *demand* for health care. Thus, they restrict the *supply* of health care: restricting access to specialists, reducing the number of medical graduates, closing hospital beds, deinsuring certain services, capping physician income, limiting the use of modern equipment—the list stretches on.

At some level, it makes sense. Doctors are expensive to train and costly to pay. Cut the number of medical graduates and cap the income of those in practice, and you save money. High-tech equipment costs money to buy and maintain. Hold back on purchasing and utilization of diagnostic equipment, and you save. There's just one catch: what if you happen to be a patient?

The insanity of the situation was well illustrated when, in the late 1990s, several British Columbian physicians publicly protested the lengthy waiting list for MRIs on Vancouver Island. With a population of over 600,000 people, the island had only one MRI machine. To make matters worse, the scanner was allowed to operate only on bankers' hours, being mandated to perform no more than 3,000 scans per year. The end result was a year-long waiting time for an "elective" MRI. But this term is deceptive. One patient on the waiting list, for example, was suspected of having an acoustic neuroma, a slow-growing cancer. For months, she waited, every day wondering if cancer was growing in her head. Patients suspected of having multiple sclerosis were also forced to wait. Imagine the sword of MS hanging over your head for a year. In an ironic twist, provincial regulations require that MS patients, in order to receive certain drug therapies, must first have the disease confirmed by an MRI scan.

Therein lies the dirty truth of Canadian health care. It is just like the old Soviet system: everything is free, but nothing is readily available. It may be entertaining to talk about people queuing for toilet paper in Moscow in the 1970s. It's far less funny to think about a Canadian with MS waiting for an MRI today.

British and European Health Care

Proponents of government-run health care tend to look beyond Canada when they cite a potential model for the United States. European systems now serve the role that Canada's once did.[13] But while the woes of these systems are less appreciated in the United States, public health care is anything but a success story in Europe.

Britain's NHS may be the most plagiarized health-care system in the Western world—decades ago, it was the British model that served as the inspiration for politicians in Sweden, Canada, Australia, and New Zealand. These days, Britain's NHS doesn't seem like much of a model for anything—except, perhaps, frustration.

Margaret Dixon's care is a case in point. An English pensioner awaiting a risky surgery, she was prepped for the procedure and, expecting the worst, said goodbye to her family—only to be bumped by a more urgent case. Again she waited, again she was prepped, and again she said goodbye to her family—and she was bumped again. In all, she says, her surgery has been canceled seven times. (National Health Service officials dispute her account, arguing it's "only" been four times.)

Ms. Dixon's problems aren't isolated. Consider that Britain's NHS has roughly a million people waiting for care and that 200,000 wait longer than six months. So overstretched is the system that horror stories litter British papers: the time a woman died from cancer when her surgery was delayed several times; the incident when a hospital chapel was used as a makeshift morgue; the questionable care of a 94-year-old woman who was found by her family still in the emergency ward, unwashed and agitated, three days after arriving to the hospital. The latter drew the fiercest response from NHS officials, who maintained that they had done nothing wrong—and promptly released confidential patient information in an effort to bolster their case.

Continental systems are no less problematic. True, the French run circles around the English—decision making is more decentralized; little distinction is made between public and private facilities (allowing patients choice); modest user fees are charged, cutting down on some frivolous expenses; care is timely. French medicine is also quirky. For instance, patients can refer themselves to specialists—it's seen as a right.[14] But the over-reaching hand of government is felt everywhere. A majority of hospitals, including the country's largest, are state-owned. Philippe Manière, editor of the French business and economics journal *L'Expansion,* describes the situation:

> Mismanagement and waste compound the burden of the health care system. The majority of France's state-owned hospitals are managed in a way that is reminiscent of the old U.S.S.R. For example, in the average French public hospital, it is not uncommon for every window to be open, even in winter, because the heating system for the building cannot be regulated. With the only options being no heat or unbearably high heat, everyone opts for the latter. Predictably, this is not very cheap.[15]

Standards of care can be lax. A hot summer in 2003 led to death by dehydration for nearly 15,000 elderly people because physicians were on vacation and hospitals were slow to react (and, on top of everything, generally lacked air conditioning systems).

Percentage of Patients Having to Wait More Than 4 Months for Non-Emergency Surgery[16]

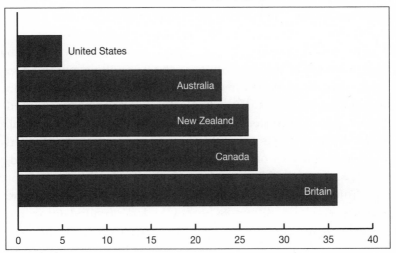

Source: Commonwealth Fund

Use of High-Tech Medical Procedures (per 100,000 per year)[17]

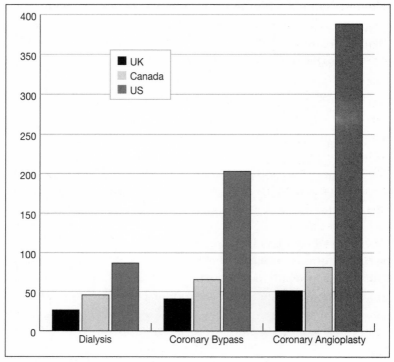

Source: *Health Affairs*

If French health care appears shaky, the house of German health care sinks on its unsustainable foundation. "The German health care system is facing bankruptcy on an unprecedented level," states the *Lancet,* the prestigious British medical journal. Faced with rising pressures, the German government has looked to various methods of cost containment, such as global spending caps. One colorful result: large-scale doctor strikes.

Some say the quality of care suffers. "Not even half the patients who have suffered a heart attack are treated according to the medical state-of-art," observes Ulla Schmidt. "Health care for women—especially precautions against breast cancer—is so bad that it results in unnecessary amputations and late diagnosis."[18] This is a compelling statement coming from a former federal minister for health and social security.

Other countries suffer similar woes. In fact, there are clear patterns that can be seen across these very different systems: decisions are colored by politicization, bureaucratization, and a disdain of innovation.

Politicization. There's a British expression that whenever a bedpan falls in England, it rings in Parliament—every detail, no matter how small, gets noticed in the chambers of power, inevitably leading to a politicization of every decision. In the Canadian province of Saskatchewan, for example, politicians closed "redundant" rural hospitals but found no need to touch those in urban areas—where their voters live. In France, the government pays for a popular, if scientifically unproven, remedy for "heavy legs."

Bureaucratization. With so much money involved, it's inevitable that bureaucratic rules are drafted to control and influence spending. In the mid-1990s, Ontario hospitals pined to get CAT scanners while health bureaucrats worried about the cost. At a meeting of senior bureaucrats, the deputy minister pointed to a photocopier in the corner of the office and asked, "What would you say if I told you that the Ministry of Health should have a committee established to determine if each office should be allowed to get a machine and under what circumstance?" Actually, such a committee already existed.

Anti-Innovation. In his classic analysis of political entrepreneurship, *An Overgoverned Society,* the economist W. Allen Wallis noted that politicians compete for votes by offering new government services.[19] Drawing on Wallis's theory of political entrepreneurship, the Nobel laureate economist Milton Friedman recently observed that "once the bulk of costs have been taken over by government ... the political entrepreneur has no additional groups to attract, and attention turns to holding down costs."[20] For this reason, public health-care systems have an inherent bias against updating services and procedures. Thus, in countries like Canada, medical technology lags behind the United States.

Availability of Medical Technology in British Columbia (Canada), Washington State, and Oregon Hospitals[21]

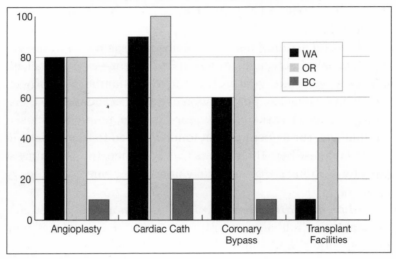

Source: Fraser Institute

Isn't it better in a public system?

European systems have major problems. But then, so does American health care. How do the former stack up against the latter? Paul Krugman wrote extensively on this issue in 2005. Like many single-payer advocates, he argues that American health care is inferior to other systems:

> Americans tend to believe that we have the best health care system in the world.... But it isn't true. We spend far more per person on health care ... yet rank near the bottom among industrial countries in indicators from life expectancy to infant mortality.[22]

Krugman makes a common error: assuming that health insurance and health go hand in hand.

But life is not so simple. Take infant mortality: according to the National Center for Health Statistics, Mexican American and white babies in the United States have the lowest infant mortality rates (about 6 in 1,000 live births), compared with Native

Americans (9) and blacks (14). Yet Mexican Americans have the least access to health insurance of these groups. In fact, it's even more complicated: a study in the *Journal of the American Medical Association* suggests that Mexican American babies are twice as likely to be born outside a hospital as babies of other groups.[23]

Infant mortality statistics—like life expectancy—reflect a mosaic of factors, such as parental diet, marital status, drug use, and cultural values. So judging American health care only by such statistics is like declaring Cuban democracy stronger than America's based on voter turnout.

Krugman argues that health care in the United States, as compared with other industrialized countries, isn't worth what we spend on it:

> Amazing, isn't it? U.S. health care is so expensive that our government spends more on health care than the governments of other advanced countries, even though the private sector pays a far higher share of the bills. . . . What do we get for all that money? Not much.[24]

Actually, if we measure a health-care system by how well it serves the sick, American medicine excels. Consider the following cancer studies:

• Women who get breast cancer in Europe are four times as likely to be diagnosed after the tumor has spread and are less likely to survive the disease than women in the United States. Comparing breast cancer statistics in Germany, Britain, France, Spain, Italy, and the United States, the market analyst Datamonitor finds that 95 percent of American women tend to be diagnosed early, in stages I or II. By contrast, 80 percent of European women are diagnosed at these stages.[25]

• Cancer patients in the United States have markedly higher survival rates than their European counterparts. In a sweeping analysis, Datamonitor looks at cancer survival in the European Union, the United Kingdom, and the United States. For patients diagnosed with stage I colorectal cancer, survival is 90 percent in the U.S., compared with 80 percent in Germany and 70 percent in Britain. The survival rate for first-stage breast cancer is 97 percent in the U.S., but only 78 percent in Britain. Datamonitor also finds that patients tend to be diagnosed earlier in the U.S. For example, a full 70 percent of prostate cancers are caught in the early stages here, but only 58 percent are in Britain.

• The World Health Organization, in partnership with the International Union Against Cancer, compiles five-year survival rates for various types of cancers. The United States consistently bests Europe. For leukemia, the American survival rate is almost 50 percent; the European rate, 35 percent. Five-year rates for esophageal carcinoma are 12 percent in the U.S. but just 6 percent across the Atlantic.[26]

Other cancer studies replicate these results (see graphs). In other areas of medicine, the results are similar (e.g., the previously mentioned Heart and Stroke Foundation of Canada study).

Breast Cancer Mortality Ratio (those who succumb to the disease divided by those diagnosed)[27]

Source: Commonwealth Fund

Why do American patients fare so much better than their European or Canadian counterparts? There are several reasons: access to physicians and specialists, aggressiveness of treatment,

Prostate Cancer Mortality Ratio (those who succumb to the disease divided by those diagnosed)[28]

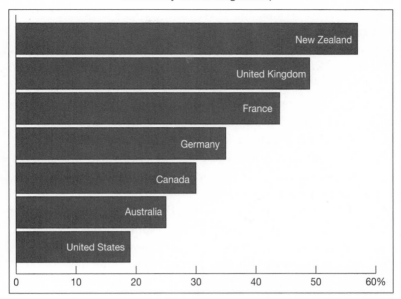

Source: Commonwealth Fund

Percentage of Patients Spending
More Than 20 Minutes with Their Doctor[29]

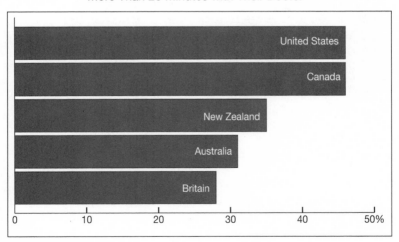

Source: *Health Affairs*

use of new technology and pharmaceuticals. In Britain, for example, it's been estimated that about 40 percent of cancer patients are not seen by an oncologist. Taxol, a medication used to treat advanced breast cancer and refractory ovarian cancer, was approved for use in Europe in 1995, but didn't reach British cancer patients until 2000.

Prof. Oliver Schöffski, director of Health Management at the University of Erlangen-Nuremberg, studies the use of pharmaceuticals in Europe. In a widely cited paper, which incorporates nearly two hundred studies, he looks at the treatment of twenty illnesses across Europe and finds a consistent pattern of underuse.[30]

As a psychiatrist, I have been particularly struck by Prof. Schöffski's analysis of antidepressants. In the United States, the first-line treatment for depression is the newer medications, the SSRIs (Prozac and her sister drugs). The older drugs are equally effective, but heavy in side effects and easy to overdose on—a serious concern when so many depressed patients have suicidal ideations. Thus, the newer medications are clearly superior to the old ones. Prof. Schöffski finds that only one-third of German patients who are treated for depression get Prozac or the other newer meds; the majority are treated with the best pharmacology that the 1970s had to offer.[31]

The issue isn't slow drug approvals—the EU takes roughly as long as the FDA to approve new drugs.[32] Rather, the problem is the one outlined by Allen Wallis: bureaucrats eager to tighten budgets see new drugs only as new expenses, even if they save lives.

If health care is so inferior in Canada and Europe, why isn't there a push for change? Actually, there is.

Public Systems, Market Reforms

On June 9, 2005, the Supreme Court of Canada called the health-care system dangerous and deadly, striking down key laws and turning the country's vaunted medicare on its head. The ruling aptly symbolizes the declining enthusiasm for socialized medicine even in socialist countries.

The Supreme Court of Canada is arguably the most liberal high court in the Western world, having recently endorsed the constitutionality of gay marriage and the right of all prisoners to vote. Most legal scholars expressed surprise that the justices even agreed to hear this appeal of a health-care case twice dismissed by lower courts. Involving a man who waited almost a year for a hip replacement, the bench decided that the province of Quebec has no right to restrict the freedom of a person to purchase health care or health insurance. In doing so, they struck down two Quebec laws, overturning a thirty-year ban on private medicine in the province. The wording of the ruling, though, has implications beyond Quebec and could be used to scrap other major parts of Canada's federal health-care legislation.

The decision was an earthquake—call it the hip that changed health-care history.[33]

This outcome would not have been possible without the persistence of one man: Jacques Chaoulli. A Montreal physician, Chaoulli was so angered when a government bureaucrat shut down his private family practice that he went on a hunger strike. After a month, he gave up and decided that only the courts could help his fight. With an eye on a legal challenge, Chaoulli tried his hand at law school, but flunked out after a semester. Undeterred, he sought the help of various organizations to support his efforts. None would. He decided to proceed anyway, choosing to represent himself. His legal fight, costing more than a half million dollars, was funded largely by his Japanese father-in-law.

The Supreme Court of Canada's decision legitimizes a trend: more than ever, Canadians look to private medicine. In Quebec, the government announced plans to contract out surgeries for knee and hip replacements to the private sector. The Alberta and British Columbia governments are weighing similar measures.

Dr. Brian Day's clinic flourishes—and it's in good company. Hip replacements can now be purchased in private Quebec clinics. Prominent American hospitals, like the M. D. Anderson Cancer Center and the Cleveland Clinic, boast offices in Toronto, encouraging Canadians to access their services. And medical brokers like Timely Medical Alternatives will offer Canadians options for wait-free care on both sides of the 49th parallel.

While Canadian governments look to market reforms, similar changes are occurring under Britain's Labour government.

It didn't start out that way in Tony Blair's administration. On the day before his election as prime minister in 1997, he declared: "Twenty-four hours to save the NHS!" Blair's vision for the NHS was profoundly hostile to markets. He pledged to banish the (modest) internal competition introduced by Margaret Thatcher, scrap the deals between private insurance companies and the NHS, and cut down on private medicine by cutting down on the need for it.

But then a funny thing happened on the way to saving the NHS. It didn't get better. Indeed, despite the centralization and the funding increases, Blair's government endured a host of problems: long waiting lists, public anger, overcrowded emergency rooms—especially during a flu outbreak one winter. That changed opinion at 10 Downing Street. The government inked a five-page document and called it *For the Benefit of Patients.* Never before has such a revolutionary paper gone out under such an uninspired title. The document begins: "There should be no organisational or ideological barriers to the delivery of high quality health care free at the point of delivery to those who need it."[34]

In their election manifesto of 2005, Labour promised to triple the number of surgeries provided by the private sector—from 5 percent of all non-emergency procedures to 15 percent in 2008. The Labour government now works to voucherize certain surgeries, offering patients a choice of four providers, at least one of which is private. Needless to say, the independent sector is thriving.[35]

Other countries also look to market reforms:

• To encourage citizens to buy private insurance, the Australian government offers tax subsidies for private health care and even financial penalties for wealthier citizens who stay in the public system. Enrollment in private plans approaches 45 percent of the population.[36]

• Facing spiraling costs, the Stockholm City Council began privatizations in the mid-1990s: home care, ambulance services, and diagnostic testing. Laboratory costs fell by 30 percent; support staff costs, by 30 percent; ambulance costs, by 15 percent.[37]

The council also ended restrictions on primary care. Today, Stockholm's reforms continue, surviving three changes in government. After the completion of the latest round of privatizations, some 80 percent of Stockholm's primary care and 40 percent of total health services will be contracted out. Privatization has not been limited to just these services. In 1999, St. George's Hospital, one of Stockholm's largest, was sold to Capio Ltd., a private company.

• In the mid-1990s, South Africa's Mandela government sought to encourage citizens to opt for private insurance. To this end, South Africa deregulated the insurance market, creating perhaps the most unfettered market for private insurance in the world. Plans along the lines of a health savings account are the most popular.

• Finland sees privatization and contracting out as a major tool in the reform of public services. Since 1995, municipalities have been allowed to buy services from the private sector. Whereas in 1989 the public sector employed some 215,000 people, by 1996 this number was down to 127,000.[38] In the area of health and welfare, contracting out has become commonplace. One municipality recently went so far as to privatize all of its health provision.

• Recent German reforms—started by the Red-Green coalition—mean that patients must pay small fees when they visit a doctor or fill a prescription, and that private insurers are given a more prominent role. The initiative builds on earlier reforms that will put the vast majority of German hospitals in private hands. By 2015, only a few hundred of Germany's 1,700 hospitals will remain under the control of the state.[39]

• Several countries with social insurance–style health care—including Belgium, the Netherlands, and the Czech Republic—encourage modest competition among the different insurers.[40]

All these trends need to be kept in perspective, of course. Market reforms are increasingly under consideration in countries like Canada, but so are a host of other ideas. Like an alcoholic slipping back into his habit, governments tend to latch onto central-planning schemes. The Blair government, for example, has been open-minded about contracting out to the independent sector, but has also pushed ahead with a variety of initiatives that aren't exactly market-oriented, like NICE, a euphemistically named committee whose role is to contain prescription drug costs by effectively dictating to physicians the types and amounts of medications they ought to be prescribing.

John Martin, the director of Employment, Labour and Social Affairs at the Organisation for Economic Co-operation and Development, notices various approaches employed by governments with public systems to contain health costs. Testifying before Congress, he said that "cost-efficiency oriented reforms"—such as decentralizing decision making and introducing greater competition among providers—can be seen in numerous countries.[41] But he is quick to point out that other strategies for holding down costs, like price controls and budget caps, have also been implemented in these countries.

Still, the ideological shift has been profound. Political systems are slow to change, being weighed down by interest-group demands, union obstruction, and public angst. Politicized health care is no different. But the direction of change is clear: toward a market orientation, away from central planning. American academics may rhapsodize about the triumph of socialist health care in other countries. But in the streets of Stockholm and London, it's the ideas of Adam Smith that percolate.

TEN

The Three Keys

ON A SNOWY NIGHT IN March 2005, citizens packed into a large
room of the capitol in Montpelier, Vermont, to hear me debate
Dr. Deborah Richter, a family physician, on the topic of a single-
payer health-care system. It's difficult not to admire Dr. Richter
for the boldness of her position. Nationally, single-payer fell out
of fashion with the demise of HillaryCare. Even in Vermont, the
land of Howard Dean and Ben & Jerry's, the idea holds purchase
only with a handful of state legislators. Yet despite all this, Dr.
Richter energetically tours the state calling for a single-payer system—not watered-down half measures like an expansion of
Medicare to cover those over 55, not a new federal drug discount
card, but a full-out single-payer system. Standing at the lectern,
listening to her talk about pushing ourselves to imagine a different kind of American health care, I thought: we must do that.

The reforms I've advocated so far have been pragmatic, aiming to improve American health care today. Most of the major
ideas have been supported by both Republicans and Democrats
at one time or another, and could be implemented right now. The
most controversial of these ideas—modeling Medicare after the
Federal Employee Health Benefits Plan—was the chief recommendation of the Breaux-Thomas Bipartisan Commission on the
Future of Medicare. All of these ideas are ways of optimizing components of the system now in place.

Can we think bigger—outside the proverbial box? Need we
be wedded to our current health-care system and all its parts?

Are there more fundamental changes that could instill more choice and competition?

I believe that we can bring about more basic change in three key areas. First, we can make health care portable. Second, we can rethink how to provide health care to the elderly. Finally, we can create a market that will catalyze innovation in drugs and medical devices. In these areas, we can build on the thinking of Milton Friedman, Wilbur Mills, and Gary Becker, respectively. Doing so will allow us to unlock the hidden potential of American health care.

Making Health Insurance Portable

I recently asked a friend in New York about her job and she seemed to have everything—a good salary, excellent benefits, a great view from her office. There's just one problem: "I hate my job," she says. A lawyer by training, she's been working as a book editor for a couple of years. She would love to quit and write a book on a technical aspect of law. But if she leaves her job, she isn't sure she could afford health insurance for her family.

My friend happens to live in New York City, where health insurance is expensive—costing perhaps five or six times more than in cities like Columbus and Sacramento. She wonders what life might be like with a Canadian-style system. "I wouldn't need to worry about premiums," she reflects. She's trapped by the system of employer-sponsored insurance. Her job is a vehicle to get health care as much as to make money.

With rising costs, employers also worry. In the fall of 2005, a confidential memo leaked from Wal-Mart offered a window on employers' strategies to contain premium costs. The memo, prepared for the board of directors, recommended: "Given the significant savings from even a small improvement in the health of our Associate base, Wal-Mart should seek to attract a healthier workforce.... A healthier workforce will lead to lower health insurance costs, lower absenteeism through fewer sick days, and higher productivity."[1] The memo outlined several ideas, including: "Design all jobs to include some physical activities."

While Wal-Mart is trying to reduce the financial burden of benefits, other companies are dropping coverage altogether. In the last five years, the percentage of employers offering health coverage has dropped 9 percent. Providing benefits is no longer such a good deal for employers, because the world that gave birth to this system no longer exists.

As we have seen, employer-sponsored insurance rose out of the wage and price controls of the Second World War. At that time, health care was cheap, and many stayed with the same employer for their working lives. In the era of the company town, complete with the company swimming club, the company health plan made sense. Under a generous tax incentive, this coverage grew. Between 1939 and 1945, employer-sponsored health insurance went from the exception to the emerging standard, up from 8 percent of the American population to 25 percent.[2]

But the company town and the employer-for-life are nearly extinct. Today's workforce is more mobile. The typical employee stays at a small or midsized company for eighteen months; people frequently change their jobs (though less so among larger employers). That has wide-ranging repercussions for a health-care system built on employer-sponsored insurance. Among the most unfortunate consequences is that as people leave jobs, they lose their insurance.

We can make it easier for Americans to obtain and keep health insurance. Consumer-driven health plans—and, in particular, health savings accounts—can provide lower-cost insurance, without the paternalism of managed care. (The Wal-Mart memo, for instance, calls for HSAs.) For those between jobs, we can expand the health tax exclusion to cover non-employer purchases of health insurance; individuals could then deduct the cost of premiums from their taxes. The present tax code rewards employers and penalizes employees. By expanding deductibility, Congress could achieve a more equitable dynamic, at relatively modest cost to the Treasury.

But is this really the best approach? After all, it would only serve as a band-aid, providing some tax relief to people who are self-employed or between jobs. It could be opposed on the grounds that expanding the tax exclusion would merely expand the tax insanity.

That's the view of Milton Friedman, who has spent decades contemplating the economic problems of American health care. In the course of writing this book, I asked him what he would do to better the system. He told me that Congress should reconsider the whole notion of a health tax exclusion.

> There is no more reason for an employer to provide his employees with medical care than there is for him to provide them with food or clothing or housing. The reason why employer provided medical care is so prevalent today is a result of a tax provision introduced during and following World War II which exempted employer financed medical care from taxes. This loophole in the tax system has done tremendous harm. It has caused the medical care industry to develop in an inefficient and unnatural way.
>   The best reform would be to eliminate the tax deduction of any medical care expenses. There is no more reason for medical care expenses to be tax deductible than for food, clothing, and housing expenses to be tax deductible. A minimum deduction for all of them is provided in the personal exemption.[3]

Eliminating the tax deduction would, of course, mean more tax revenue. Employer-based health coverage costs Washington dearly. Based on calculations by John Sheils and Randall Haught, both of the Lewin Group, tax-free health insurance cost nearly $200 billion in 2004—more, incidentally, than the tax subsidy for mortgages.

Some have looked at that number and seen a potential boon in federal tax revenue. They ponder how to divide up the bounty— like a family standing over the Thanksgiving turkey. A *New York Times* essay, for example, extolled the virtues of using the money to insure all the uninsured.[4] From this vantage point, ending the exclusion seems like finding new money without any budgetary sacrifice.

But that's not quite correct. For millions of Americans, particularly those in higher tax brackets, ending the exclusion would mean a major tax hike—even if most opted for less expensive insurance. In the real world, therefore, it is unlikely that this large and powerful voting block would accept such a change without some sort of compensatory tax reform.[5]

More to the point, if employers aren't given an incentive to offer health insurance, many will stop providing these benefits. Where then would Americans get their insurance?

The question may seem daunting, but the answer that Prof. Friedman suggests is actually quite simple. Americans can get their insurance the good old-fashioned way: through the free market. Health insurance can be purchased directly by the individual or his family.

What would health insurance look like in a non-employer-sponsored system?

First, without the tax exclusion, people would choose higher deductibles in their health insurance—which would then move away from its present, all-encompassing definition. People typically buy insurance for an unforeseen or unlikely event; but with minimal deductibles, health insurance has effectively become a form of prepaid health care. Faced with the high cost of comprehensive insurance, most Americans would probably do what they do when they buy, say, home insurance: choose a higher deductible. Not only would this end the overinsurance problem as people became price-conscious health consumers, but even older individuals would be able to find more affordable premiums.

Second, if Congress and state legislatures loosened regulations on health insurance, new players would emerge quickly: charities, associations, and unions would start offering health insurance. Instead of getting their health insurance from their employers, people might opt to buy a policy through their church or synagogue. It's also possible that companies would market options. Just as Templeton offers mutual funds and Barclays sells exchange-traded funds to address America's need for financial vehicles, companies would offer Americans different insurance options if they joined a common pool.

The experience of the Federal Employee Health Benefits Plan suggests that, offered choices and reasonable prices, people are willing to join a larger pool, even if it means paying slightly higher premiums. With nine million participants, the FEHBP is quite a big pool; but it's easy to see that, say, an AFL-CIO insurance pool could be just as large.

Third, aware of the premiums rising with age, insurance companies would offer options like guaranteed renewability, allowing younger people to "lock in" their rates.

There is still a minority of people who would be difficult to insure. Low in income, high in risk, these individuals could use a helping hand. Assuming that charity pools weren't available, there may then be a need for states to expand existing high-risk pools (that is, programs for high-risk people to buy private insurance at lower rates). But for the vast majority of Americans, individual insurance would work well.

This may not seem like a practical solution at present. While employer-sponsored health insurance has few enthusiastic advocates, individual insurance draws many critics. Two principle objections can be made, both amounting to the accusation that such a system would be unfair. First, there would be a huge variation in premiums across states. A resident of New York City, where a basic plan is unaffordable to many, could take a train to Connecticut and the same policy would cost 75 percent less. Second, without significant government intervention, such a system would discriminate against those who need health care most. Because the present risk-pooling would be lost, the executive assistant with a heart condition couldn't get insurance—potentially only the wealthy and healthy could.

There are answers to these criticisms, however. State variation need not be permanent. The fundamental problem isn't so much the market as the regulation of the individual market. New York—where even podiatry must be covered by insurance plans—is a case in point. We need to make the market work better, not abandon it. Congress can enforce the commerce clause of the Constitution by creating a national market for health insurance.

As for penalizing the unhealthy, the magnitude of the problem is almost certainly overstated. Even the claim that chronically ill Americans consume the vast majority of health resources needs some refinement. It's true that a small number of people consume a disproportionately large amount of health care. In 1996, for instance, 1 percent of health-care users accounted for

28 percent of expenses.[6] The top 5 percent used 56 percent and the top 10 percent used 70 percent. But how many of that costly 1 percent actually stayed in that high-expense category the following year? Relatively few—only about one in seven.[7] Moreover, the market would almost surely rise to the challenge, offering different types of pools (through churches, for example) and more consumer options.

In short, many often-expressed concerns about individual insurance are unfounded or misplaced. Americans want portability in health insurance and freedom of labor movement—yet they are saddled with a tax code that rewards a 1940s ideal of health insurance. It's time to update the code, and help create portable insurance along the way.

Shoring up Medicare

To my great despair, my daughter Emma swims in debt. She owes nearly $28,000—and her debts are accumulating quickly. Emma, though, isn't a gambler or a compulsive shopper. She's just an infant and can barely walk. Her debt problems don't flow from bad choices she has made, but rather from poor decisions that political leaders made before her birth. But if Emma is now deeply in debt, the future is even more worrisome: Medicare threatens to add substantially to the national debt (and her personal share of it) or cripple her economic future with high taxes—or both. Something must be done.

Though Social Security has recently received the most attention, it's only one of three major federal social expenditures. Medicare ultimately poses more of a threat. In one of his last addresses as chairman of the Federal Reserve, Alan Greenspan reviewed the numbers:

> In fiscal year 2005, federal outlays for Social Security, Medicare, and Medicaid totaled about 8 percent of gross domestic product. The long-run projections from the Office of Management and Budget suggest that the share will rise to 9.5 percent by 2015 and to about 13 percent by 2030. So long as health-care costs continue to grow faster than the economy as a whole, they will exert budget pressures that seem increasingly likely to make current fiscal policy unsustainable.[8]

Medicaid grows, as we have seen, because the scope of the program has expanded so dramatically in recent years. But Social Security and Medicare suffer from another malady: the aging of the population. Medicare is now a pay-as-you-go system—the money flows in from today's taxpayers, funding today's beneficiaries. That was fine back in the early days of Medicare, when the median age of the population was roughly 25. Today it pushes 40, and the aging continues. In 2008, the first of the baby boomers will reach 62, allowing them to begin drawing Social Security. Three short years later, they will qualify for Medicare.[9]

This means that Medicare is on shaky ground. First, as the number of beneficiaries soars, the burden on Medicare will grow as well, causing enormous future debt. (In 2005, Medicare required a transfer of roughly 9 percent of federal revenue.) Second, because money is spent, not invested, trillions of dollars worth of capital will be lost to the economy. Finally, as Medicare costs rise, Washington will attempt to hold the line on expenditures through wage and price controls—essentially shifting the costs to private plans.

A major step in shoring up Medicare will involve returning to Wilbur Mills' original vision of the program. He saw at the outset that a pay-as-you-go system was unsustainable. Speaking to the Arkansas-Missouri District Kiwanis Convention in September 1964 about an early version of the Medicare bill, he warned:

> In practical terms, this meant that if the hospital insurance system which would be created by the bill was to remain sound, the taxable wage base would have to be increased at least $150 each year. Clearly, this would be a case of the tail wagging the dog. The Congress would be left completely hamstrung, with only two alternatives: (1) A total program which we know was actuarially unsound, or (2) a commitment into the indefinite future to a steady but wholly uncontrolled increase, due to the hospital part of the program, in the amount of wages taxed for social security purposes. Clearly, we could not conscientiously be a party to such an abrogation of congressional responsibility.[10]

In an earlier speech, Mills suggested some type of prefunding of Medicare to make it sustainable. "I would be hopeful," he said, "that the prepayment concept might lead us in the direction of sound approaches on this matter."[11]

The arguments for prefunding Medicare are similar to those advanced for prefunding Social Security. We know that the future obligations of Medicare will be astronomical. If we can put away money over the coming decade and allow the capital to accrue interest, the final liability will be more manageable. The principle is a sound one. At an individual level, for instance, a person saving just a thousand dollars a year for forty years at a 7 percent return would have nearly a quarter of a million dollars. That is my approach to saving for my daughter Emma's college years, and it offers a good model for how we as a nation can cover her future medical expenses.

How would this work in practice? Some have suggested that, in the spirit of the collective nature of Medicare, the prefunding be done on a collective basis. Prof. Laurence Seidman (University of Delaware) argues in *Health Affairs* that the federal government should set aside money in a new, designated trust fund, complete with its own commissioner. For those familiar with the history of Social Security, though, this idea seems less than compelling. Back in the early 1980s, a commission made exactly such a recommendation and Congress acted upon it. According to Alan Greenspan, who chaired the commission, this has not been a success:

> Unfortunately, the current Social Security system has not proven a reliable vehicle for such saving. Indeed, although the trust funds have been running annual surpluses since the mid-1980s, one can credibly argue that they have served primarily to facilitate larger deficits in the rest of the budget and therefore have added little or nothing to national saving.[12]

In other words, a new trust fund for Medicare is unlikely to get us further ahead.

A better approach would be to personalize the savings. There would be some options:

- Set aside part of the payroll tax into registered health accounts, to be invested in stocks and bonds over the beneficiaries' working lives.

- Set aside part of general revenue into special accounts, invested over time, then paid out to beneficiaries.
- Expand present savings options, like Roth IRAs.

There are some problems with the concept of prefunding. If today's workers are saving for their own Medicare futures, what of today's beneficiaries? There is a significant transitional cost. For just this reason, much of the Social Security debate is bogged down in arguments about the size of the transition and its funding. For critics of private accounts for Social Security, the certain burden of transition would be shouldered without any certainty of future gain.

Prefunding Medicare is not the same as prefunding Social Security. For one thing, the financial outlook of Medicare is significantly worse. For another, the much larger capital infusion created by private accounts—four to five times the infusion that would be created by private Social Security accounts—would reduce the volatility of the investment. But precisely because the amount of money required to pre-fund Medicare is so much larger, it would be a massive effort.[13] On this score, since predicting future pension spending is far easier than estimating future medical costs, the Social Security debate is miles ahead of any rethinking of Medicare. Most estimates are based on past health spending, but the past is not necessarily predictive of the future.

Before any serious weighing of how to prefund, the program itself needs serious reconsideration. Medicare is flawed not simply in its long-term outlook, but in its basic structure (problems that are, of course, interrelated). Earlier, we looked at the idea of moving away from the present zero-dollar structure, toward some type of premium-support model. In conjunction with this, we should rethink the scope of Medicare. At present, it covers all Americans who reach their 65th birthday—a requirement unchanged since 1965, even though people now live longer and healthier. Medicare could become more solvent by raising the age of eligibility, as Social Security has done.

Here, then, is a plan for reforming Medicare. First, as I argued in Chapter Seven, we need to move the debate back to 1999, when a bipartisan commission agreed that the program needs to be replaced by competing private plans. Second, Congress should allow Americans to prefund the medical care of their twilight years. Finally, Congress must reconsider the age of eligibility.

Creating a Market for Medical Progress

The best way to appreciate the limits of modern medicine is to practice it. In my clinical experience, people like my patient Michael illustrate the serious limitations of my profession.

Luck would seem to have favored Michael. His father was a wealthy businessman who could afford the best for his son. Michael went to an exclusive high school, summered in France, and owned a cool car even before he had a license. He was different from other teenagers.

Material wealth wasn't the only difference. Around age seventeen, Michael became increasingly disorganized. Previously a good student, he slept through classes and failed to produce assignments on time. His family doctor wondered about depression. But soon the diagnosis declared itself fully, when he developed paranoid thoughts. He worried that family members were conspiring against him, poisoning his food, tapping his phone. Psychotic and agitated, he was admitted to a hospital for the first of many times.

Making the diagnosis was easy—Michael clearly had schizophrenia—but the treatment would prove challenging. He developed strong side effects on risperidone, a new antipsychotic. He disliked the weight gain of olanzapine. For years he went without medications, eventually living on the street on the West Coast.

When I saw Michael, I started a trial of clozapine. He did amazingly well. His paranoia abated. His disorganized thoughts grew logical. But then he developed a cardiac side effect, and we were back to square one.

Despite the incredible advances of the past decades, doctors still face limitations. In my practice of psychiatry, I feel these limits daily, especially in my inability to help so many with schizophrenia. Doctors in other fields are just as frustrated. Our treatment of strokes can now help limit the damage, but can't undo it. Treatments for Alzheimer's barely best placebos, despite more than a century of research. Yet if we can all agree on the importance of developing better medications, practically no one is willing to do anything to address a major roadblock to their development.

In Chapter Eight, we considered the problems with the FDA, where hyper-regulation chokes every aspect of drug development, and I proposed several solutions. The basic idea is that drugs need to come to the market faster. Gary Becker, who won the Nobel Memorial Prize in Economic Sciences in 1992, has a bold idea for achieving this goal: he would return the FDA to its original mandate.

Prof. Becker argues that the FDA should concern itself solely with safety, not with safety *and* efficacy as it does now. He suggests making efficacy testing voluntary. Drug companies could then choose whether or not to opt for this additional testing (a decision that would be disclosed to patients). Whereas today's market for pharmaceuticals is dominated by a handful of companies, dropping efficacy testing would allow drug innovation to flourish in more places. Becker explains:

> It follows that a return to a safety standard alone would lower costs and raise the number of therapeutic compounds available. In particular, this would include more drugs from small biotech firms that do not have the deep pockets to invest in extended efficacy trials. And the resulting increase in competition would mean lower prices—without the bureaucratic burden of price controls. In turn, cheaper and more diverse drugs would induce insurance companies and public providers to cover many more new drugs, even when their efficacy was uncertain.
>
> Elimination of the efficacy requirement would give patients, rather than the FDA, the ultimate responsibility of deciding which drugs to try. Presumably, the vast majority of patients would continue to rely on the opinions of physicians about which drugs to use.
>
> But many people whose lives are at risk want to believe that they ultimately make the decisions—even when they essentially follow the experts' advice.[14]

If, as Prof. Becker contends, we would gain so much by eliminating the efficacy requirement, why should we have this requirement? Regulatory bodies are usually concerned only with safety.

In car production, for instance, the government demands that GM's latest model meet certain basic safety standards—for example, in its airbags. It doesn't demand that a new Taurus make for a "good drive." Similarly, if Kellogg's wants to bring a new breakfast cereal to market, it must meet food safety regulations; but it doesn't need to show that the cereal is satisfying or filling.

In drug development, the end result of the efficacy requirement is an incredibly complex and laborious approval process. How much do the efficacy trials add to the total cost of bringing a drug to market? Probably around 40 percent. In many cases, the FDA's efficacy requirement is simply irrelevant, since drugs are often used for purposes other than the approved ones. The antibiotic amoxicillin, for instance, is approved for the treatment of respiratory illness because a drug company took it through all three phases of clinical trials to get that certification. But amoxicillin is also useful in treating a variety of conditions, including stomach ulcers; medical textbooks recommend it for this use, and doctors prescribe it accordingly. But the antibiotic hasn't gone through Phase II and Phase III trials for the treatment of ulcers, nor has it been certified for efficacy in this use. Amoxicillin for stomach ulcers is an off-label use.

Back in the 1990s, the General Accounting Office looked into off-label uses of cancer drugs. Focusing on 46 drugs and hormonal agents, the GAO studied the prescribing habits of oncologists and found that 44 of the 46 drugs were prescribed for an off-label indication. In fact, off-label prescribing appears to be the norm, not the exception, for cancer treatment. According to GAO testimony before Congress, more than half of cancer patients had at least one off-label drug as part of their chemotherapy regimen.[15]

Defenders of the efficacy testing requirement maintain that the regimen is nevertheless relevant, if for no other reason than preventing waste. Without tests to establish efficacy, they argue, drugs that do little or nothing could come to market. To this argument, Becker responds:

> To be sure, some sick individuals would try ineffective treatments that would otherwise have been prevented from reaching market under present FDA regulations. But the quantity of reliable health information now available with only a little initia-

tive is many times greater than when the efficacy standard was
introduced four decades ago. WebMD and other Internet
sources, along with better and more extensive health reporting
by the news media, offer medical consumers superior access to
information than even their doctors enjoyed not long ago.

A drug that did little or nothing would not remain on the market
for long. A drug that saved or improved lives, however, would
quickly find and keep a market share. To ensure that this happens, policymakers should remove the hurdles that make it so
hard, and so costly, to bring these drugs to market. The key to
better drug development, in short, lies not in government regulation, but in the promise of medical and pharmaceutical science.

The Cure

A few years ago, a man named Simon presented himself to an
emergency room. He was aggressive, confused, and agitated. His
family suggested that he was off his medications—he had taken
a low dose of antipsychotics for years, but had run out of pills
before a long weekend. Three days later, he lay in front of me on
a stretcher. In the hour before our unplanned meeting, he had
attacked a security guard and urinated on himself. He couldn't
even tell me his name. After a workup revealed no underlying
medical illness, I restarted his medications and admitted him to
my ward.

The next day, Simon was fine. He could speak normally and
intelligently. He told me the error of his failed compliance, and
talked about the jobs he had done in the past few years after his
diagnosis of schizophrenia. Simon's illness colored every aspect
of his life. He never held jobs beyond simple, part-time work. He
didn't marry. But before he resumed his medications, I saw the
considerably more disordered state he would have lived in just
sixty years ago. In the era before antipsychotics, Simon would
have been sent to an asylum to spend his days in chaos. Instead,
he walked out of my hospital and returned to a relatively stable
life.

We are surrounded today by medical marvels that would have seemed miraculous during World War II, when our current health-care system was created. Since then, medicine has been transformed—and the American contribution to this change cannot be understated. Even with penicillin, a British discovery, it was American industrial innovation that brought the antibiotic to medicine cabinets. In the coming years, we can expect more of the same: cures for some types of cancers, further advances in the treatment of dementia, breakthroughs in the diagnosis and management of mental illnesses. The United States will be at the forefront of these discoveries.

Yet while the good is getting better, the bad is getting worse. Despite the advances in medicine, health-care policy is wracked by what seem to be unsolvable problems. About these problems, policymakers have talked much and done little. If the 1990s were a time of vast ambition—the sweeping proposal of Hillary Clinton, the feverish state experimentation in Tennessee and beyond, the rise and fall of managed care—the first decade of the twenty-first century has been marked by quiet resignation.

After much talk of rethinking Medicare in 2003, the White House pushed through an expansion without any significant reforms. President Bush commented on rising health costs in his State of the Union address of 2006, where he called for modest tinkering with the tax code, gave passing mention to Medicaid, and largely ignored Medicare. Even that modest agenda seems beyond the capacity of Congress to act on, with legislators unable to decide on minor changes to the structure of health savings accounts. For most of 2005, the House and the Senate debated over Medicaid changes that would reduce the program's annual growth rate from 7.7 percent to 7.5 percent by 2015, but ultimately they could not agree. The dynamic isn't much different outside the Beltway. At the state level, the most exciting initiative is seen in Massachusetts—a plan heavy in subsidies and coercion, light in meaningful reform.

Proposals that question the status quo are often dismissed as "unrealistic." David Cutler, the Harvard dean and former adviser to President Clinton, once commented to me that talk of, say, ending employer-sponsored health insurance amounted to nothing more than a "purple sky discussion"—that is, a conversation about what if the sky were purple. It might be intellectually satisfying, "but the sky isn't purple." (He has taken his own message to heart: although he once helped Hillary Clinton formulate her health-care plan, his latest book calls merely for more experimentation with pay for performance.)

But if the sky remains blue, it need not remain clouded. If America can lead the world in medical innovation, it should also be able to rethink its health-care system. America has reformed other sectors of its economy that once appeared to be in crisis. In telecommunications, in banking, and in other sectors, this transformation has meant deregulation and increased reliance on market mechanisms. Health care is the exception. Is it any wonder that Americans are so dissatisfied? Could it be any clearer what must be done?

Health care stands at a crossroads. If we stay mired in an economic model from the World War II era, government's role will keep growing, costs will continue to swell, and Americans will eventually see the kind of rationing that has afflicted Canada. The corridors outside American emergency rooms will be crammed with dozens of people on stretchers—waiting, moaning, begging for treatment, smelling of urine and sweat. If, however, Americans unleash the market forces that have transformed the other five-sixths of their economy—if they choose more choice and more competition—then American health care will become cheaper, better, and more accessible for everyone.

Capitalism is not the cause of America's health-care problems. It is the cure.

Acknowledgments

I VERY MUCH APPRECIATE the support of the Manhattan Institute. The staff has been exceptional, never hesitating to help me out. I highlight the assistance of a few: David DesRosiers convinced me that I should start this project; Henry Olsen convinced me that I could finish it; and Mark Riebling ensured that I did. I also wish to thank Larry Mone, the president of the Manhattan Institute, for his confidence in me.

John Cogan, Tom Miller, and Sally Pipes looked at earlier versions of this book and provided useful comments. Several people were particularly generous with their time, helping me understand the nuances of the issues: John Goodman, David Henderson, Grace-Marie Turner, Tom Saving, Rodney Nichols, Bob Moffit, Henry Miller, and Milton Friedman. Years ago, Cynthia Ramsay taught me much about health economics. David Frum introduced me to Larry Mone—for which I am deeply in his debt.

I am grateful for the generous support provided by the John Templeton Foundation, the Ewing Marion Kauffman Foundation, and the Achelis and Bodman Foundations.

I wish to thank Encounter Books and its publisher, Roger Kimball, who was a pleasure to work with. Carol Staswick ably copy-edited the manuscript.

Finally, I want to thank my family. My father served as unofficial editor and sounding board; my mother was a constant source of encouragement. My wife, as always, was infinitely helpful (and tolerant of my distracted state). Emma is too young to remember all this, but she was there and inspired me nevertheless.

Of course, the responsibility for any errors contained herein rests with the author.

Notes

Introduction

[1] The full decision can be read at: http://www.lexum.umontreal.ca/csc-scc/en/rec/html/2005scc035.wpd.html

[2] The top ten innovations, in order, are: MRI/CT, ACE inhibitors, balloon angiography, statins, mammography, CABG surgery, H2-receptor antagonists, SSRIs, cataract extraction and lens implants, hip replacements and knee replacements. Only balloon angiography and mammography have no American ties. As an aside, Japan was the second most significant country, with partial credit for two innovations.

Chapter One: Dick Cheney's Heart

[1] As quoted in Michael Bliss, *William Osler: A Life in Medicine* (Toronto: University of Toronto Press, 1999), p. 105.

[2] James Le Fanu, *The Rise and Fall of Modern Medicine* (New York: Carroll & Graf Publishers, 1999), p. xv.

[3] Calvin Coolidge, *The Autobiography of Calvin Coolidge* (New York: J. J. Little & Ives Co., 1929), p. 190.

[4] Darryl Enos and Paul Sultan, *The Sociology of Health Care: Social, Economic and Political Perspectives* (New York: Praeger, 1977).

[5] Caroline Poplin, "Managed Care," *Wilson Quarterly,* Summer 1996, p. 15.

[6] Cardiac care had not advanced greatly when President Dwight Eisenhower suffered a heart attack in 1955: his doctors treated him with six weeks of bed rest, oxygen, and morphine for pain.

[7] Nortin M. Hadler, *The Last Well Person: How to Stay Well Despite the Health-Care System* (Montreal: McGill-Queen's University Press, 2004), p. 17.

[8] Brad Evenson, "Cardiac Care Better in U.S., Study Shows," *National Post,* February 8, 2001, p. A4.

[9] "U.S. Heart Attack Trend Less Severe," *Washington Post,* March 25, 1999, p. A18.

[10] *Advanced Cardiac Life Support,* American Heart Association, 1997, pp. 1–49.

[11] In today's dollars, health spending per capita was about $500 a year.

[12] David Cutler, personal communication, November 29, 2004.

[13] In a 2002 paper, for example, the Yale economist William Nordhaus argues that the value of the increased longevity over the past century could be as large as the value of growth in all goods and services over the same period. "It would suggest that the image of a stupendously wasteful health care system is far off the mark."

Chapter Two: Two Days That Changed Health Care

[1] 433CCCH, Federal Tax Service, paragraph 6587. Federal government policy first influenced the formation of employment-based health insurance in a 1942 ruling by the War Labor Board that allowed employers to bypass wage controls during World War II by providing fringe benefits to attract workers.

[2] David Henderson, "Myths about U.S. Health Care," in *Better Medicine: Reforming Canadian Health Care,* ed. David Gratzer (Montreal: ECW Press, 2002), p. 179.

[3] If the family itemizes its deductions on its federal tax form, it can deduct its state income taxes. Therefore, the family's 5% tax rate, after taking account of deductibility, is really 3.6% = (1–.28) * 5%.

[4] Henderson, "Myths about U.S. Health Care," pp. 179–80.

[5] Ibid., p. 180.

[6] Tom Miller, "How the Tax Exclusion Shaped Today's Private Health Insurance Market," Joint Economic Committee, U.S. Congress, December 17, 2003, p. 5.

[7] John Sheils and Randall Haught, "The Cost of Tax-Exempt Health Benefits in 2004," *Health Affairs,* Web exclusive, February 25, 2004, pp. 104–12; http://content.healthaffairs.org/cgi/content/full/hlthaff.w4.106v1/DC1

[8] Ibid., p. 110.

[9] Bill Thomas, "Vision for Healthcare," Speech to the National Center for Policy Analysis, Washington, D.C., February 12, 2004.

[10] Quoted by Alizon Draper and Judith Green, "Food Safety and Consumers: Constructions of Choice and Risk," *Social Policy and Administration,* vol. 36, no. 6 (December 2002), p. 610.

[11] Stephen Pollard, "The Genie of Choice: Has It Been Let Loose in Britain?" *National Review,* June 20, 2003.

[12] Prime Minister Tony Blair, "Progress and Justice in the 21st Century," Speech to the Fabian Society, June 17, 2003.

[13] Paul Starr, *The Social Transformation of Medicine* (New York: Basic Books, 1982), p. 269.

[14] President Lyndon Johnson said at the event: "We wanted you to know, and we wanted the entire world to know, that we haven't forgotten who is the real daddy of Medicare."

[15] Lawrence Mirel, "We Call It Insurance, but That's Not Healthy," *Washington Post,* August 26, 2001, p. B2.

[16] Kate Sullivan, personal communication, September 2004.

[17] As quoted in Greg Scandlen, "The Pulse," *Health Care News,* January 1, 2003, http://heartland.org/Article.cfm?artId=11343

[18] Damien McCrystal, "He May Have Just Hit 90, but Milton Friedman Should Not Be Allowed to Rest on His Far from Nobel Laurels," *Observer,* September 22, 2002.

[19] Milton Friedman, personal communication, November 2003. Education is another area, incidentally, where total costs have increased, although technological advances there have been less striking.

[20] W. Michael Cox and Richard Alm, *Myths of Rich and Poor: Why We're Better Off Than We Think* (New York: Basic Books, 1999), p. 40.

[21] Kaiser Family Foundation and Health Research and Educational Trust, "Employer Health Benefits: 2005 Summary of Findings," Menlo Park, California, 2005, p. 1; http://www.kff.org/insurance/7315/sections/upload/7316.pdf

[22] Milton Friedman, "How to Cure Health Care," *Public Interest,* Winter 2001; http://www.hooverdigest.org/013/friedman

[23] Devon Herrick, "Why Are Health Costs Rising?" National Center for Policy Analysis, Dallas, Texas, Brief Analysis no. 437, May 7, 2003, p. 1.

[24] "Kaiser Health Poll Report," May/June 2003 Edition, Menlo Park, California, p. 16.

[25] Nelson Sabatini, personal communication, February 2003.

[26] As quoted to me by Prof. Friedman.

[27] The following figures and quotation are drawn from Friedman, "How to Cure Health Care."

[28] Ibid.

[29] Jonathan S. Skinner, Douglas O. Staiger, and Elliott S. Fisher, "Is Technological Change in Medicine Always Worth It? The Case of Acute Myocardial Infarction," *Health Affairs,* Web exclusive, February 7, 2006; http://content.healthaffairs.org/cgi/content/abstract/hlthaff.25.w34

Vanessa Fuhrmans, "A Radical Prescription," *Wall Street Journal,* May 10, 2004, p. R3.

31 Brent Pawlecki, personal communication, November 3, 2004.

32 Jack Mahoney, personal communication, November 3, 2004.

33 Fuhrmans, "A Radical Prescription."

34 Michael E. Porter and Elizabeth Olmsted Teisberg, "Redefining Competition in Health Care," *Harvard Business Review,* June 2004, p. 64.

35 Adapted from a similar analysis of the American health-care sector. See: John C. Goodman and Gerald L. Musgrave, *Patient Power: Solving America's Health Care Crisis* (Washington, D.C.: Cato Institute, 1992), p. 20.

36 Elliott S. Fisher et al., "The Implications of Regional Variations in Medicare Spending, Part 1: The Content, Quality, and Accessibility of Care," *Annals of Internal Medicine,* vol. 138, no. 4 (February 18, 2003), p. 273.

Chapter Three: Nixon's Revenge

1 Paul Starr, *The Social Transformation of American Medicine* (New York: Basic Books, 1982), p. 381.

2 Ibid.

3 David Dranove, *The Economic Evolution of American Health Care: From Marcus Welby to Managed Care* (Princeton, New Jersey: Princeton University Press, 2000), p. 65.

4 Ibid.

5 John Kerry, Address on January 21, 2004.

6 James C. Robinson, "From Managed Care to Consumer Health Insurance: The Rise and Fall of Aetna," *Health Affairs,* vol. 23, no. 2 (March/April 2004), p. 43.

7 See Debra A. Draper, Robert E. Hurley, Cara S. Lesser, and Bradley C. Strunk, "The Changing Face of Managed Care," *Health Affairs,* vol. 21, no. 1 (January/February 2002), pp. 11–23. Draper et al. note: "The distinction between HMO and preferred provider organization (PPO) products is becoming less clear as HMOs increasingly offer broad networks and no gatekeeper."

8 "Tracking Health Care Costs: Trends Stabilize but Remain High in 2002," Data Bulletin, Center for Studying Health System Change, Washington, D.C., June 2003.

9 Ibid.

10 Bob Herbert, "A Chance to Survive," *New York Times,* July 4, 1997, p. A19.

11 Dranove, *The Economic Evolution of American Health Care,* p. 88.

[12] "Matter of Trust: HMOs Get Little," *Managed Care,* January 2004; http://www.managedcaremag.com/archives/0401/0401.news_trust.html

[13] "Public Sees Huge Differences between Industries," Harris Poll #28, Harris Interactive, April 28, 1999; http://www.harrisinteractive.com/harris_poll/index.asp?PID=29

[14] David M. Studdert and Carole Roan Gresenz, "Appeals of Preservice Coverage Denials at 2 Health Maintenance Organizations," *Journal of the American Medical Association,* vol. 289, no. 7 (February 19, 2003), pp. 864–70.

[15] Ibid., p. 864.

[16] "Rx for the Health Care System," *Wall Street Journal,* October 8, 1998, p. A18.

[17] As quoted by John McClaughty, Testimony before the Governor's Bipartisan Commission on Health Care Availability and Affordability, State of Vermont; http://www.state.vt.us/health/commission/testimony/81.htm

[18] Alain Enthoven, personal communication, November 6, 2003.

[19] Prof. Enthoven developed this argument later in: Alain C. Enthoven and Brian Talbott, "Stanford University's Experience with Managed Competition," *Health Affairs,* vol. 23, no. 6 (November/December 2004), pp. 135–40.

Chapter Four: The Third Way

[1] Victor R. Fuchs, "More Variation in Use of Care, More Flat-of-the-Curve Medicine," *Health Affairs,* Web exclusive, October 7, 2004; http://content.healthaffairs.org/cgi/reprint/hlthaff.var.104v1

[2] Regina Herzlinger, personal communication, November 29, 2004.

[3] Ibid.

[4] John Mackey, "Consumer-Driven Health," Address to the State Policy Network, 12th Annual Meeting, October 21, 2004; http://www.worldcongress.com/news/Mackey_Transcript.pdf/

[5] John Goodman, personal communication, January 9, 2004.

[6] Greg Scandlen, personal communication, February 6, 2004.

[7] Martin Feldstein, "Health and Taxes," *Wall Street Journal,* January 19, 2004.

[8] Emily Fox of eHealthInsurance, personal correspondence, August 13, 2004.

[9] As quoted in: Steve Stanek, "A Critical Moment for Health Care in America," *Health Care News,* Heartland Institute, March 1, 2004; http://www.heartland.org/Article.cfm?artId=14519

[10] John Cogan, personal communication, June 30, 2004.

[11] Sarah Lueck, "Decisions, Decisions," *Wall Street Journal,* October 11, 2004, p. R5.

[12] Ibid.

[13] HRAs were established by an IRS ruling in 2002. Like HSAs, they combine catastrophic insurance with a tax-free account for medical purposes. The account, however, isn't "owned" by the account holder, but by the health plan. Thus, the money isn't necessarily portable from job to job or even health plan to health plan.

[14] Mackey, "Consumer-Driven Health."

[15] Ron Lieber, "New Way to Curb Medical Costs: Make Employees Feel the Sting," *Wall Street Journal,* June 23, 2004, p. A1.

[16] Hillary Rodham Clinton, "Now Can We Talk about Health Care?" *New York Times Magazine,* April 18, 2004, p. 26.

[17] Congressman Fortney "Pete" Stark, Remarks at "Prospects for Health Care Reform under Clinton," Washington, D.C., January 14, 1993.

[18] He emphasized this point in our interview of November 30, 2004. As well, see: Joseph P. Newhouse, "Consumer-Directed Health Plans and the RAND Health Insurance Experiment," *Health Affairs,* vol. 23, no. 6 (November/December 2004), pp. 107–13.

[19] Gail Shearer, "Impact of 'Consumer-Driven' Health Care on Consumers," Testimony before the Joint Economic Committee, U.S. Congress, February 25, 2004; http://jec.senate.gov/democrats/Documents/Hearings/shearertestimony25feb2004.pdf

[20] Rosemary D. Marcuss, "The Tax Treatment of Employment-Based Health Insurance," Testimony before the Committee on Finance, U.S. Senate, on April 26, 1994; http://www.cbo.gov/showdoc.cfm?index=4828&sequence=0

[21] David Cutler, personal communication, November 29, 2004. Prof. Cutler emphasizes, though, that his objections to HSAs have more to do with his concerns that they will discourage people from seeking care.

[22] Tom Miller of the Joint Economic Committee, U.S. Congress, was particularly helpful in formulating this response.

[23] Emily Fox of eHealthInsurance, personal correspondence, August 20, 2004.

[24] Tom Miller, "Driver's Ed for Backseat Drivers," *Health Affairs,* vol. 23, no. 6 (November/December 2004), p. 264.

[25] Ibid.

[26] Edwin Chen, "Bush Buys into Tax-Free Health Savings Account," *Los Angeles Times,* December 17, 2004.

[27] To date, only Florida and Arkansas have added HSAs to state plans.

[28] Federal Trade Commission and Department of Justice, *Improving Health Care: A Dose of Competition,* Washington, D.C., July 2004, ch. 8; http://www.ftc.gov/opa/2004/07/healthcarerpt.htm

[29] Charles E. Phelps, *Health Economics,* 2nd ed. (Boston: Addison-Wesley, 1997), p. 539.

[30] Markian Hawryluk, "California Emergency Departments Close Their Doors after Hemorrhaging Money," Amednews.com, March 24/31, 2003, http://www.ama-assn.org/amednews/2003/03/24/gvsd0324.htm

[31] Christopher J. Conover, "Health Care Regulation: A $169 Billion Hidden Tax," Policy Analysis no. 527, Cato Institute, October 4, 2004; http://www.cato.org/pubs/pas/pa-527es.html

[32] John F. Cogan, R. Glenn Hubbard, and Daniel P. Kessler, *Healthy, Wealthy, and Wise: Five Steps to a Better Health Care System* (Washington, D.C., and Stanford, California: AEI Press and The Hoover Institution, 2005), pp. 54–56.

[33] Merrill Matthews, "Bush's Unheralded Health Care Agenda," *Weekly Standard,* December 27, 2004, pp. 27–29.

[34] Lieber, "New Way to Curb Medical Costs."

[35] For an excellent discussion, see: David Wessel, "Time to Cure the Health-Choice Headache," *Wall Street Journal,* December 9, 2004, p. A2.

[36] Prof. Herzlinger is particularly vocal on the problems of this approach, noting that there is "no other industry in America where the suppliers can't quote their own price." She suggests that this weighs on innovation, like forcing car makers to quote prices on axles, wheels, and batteries, but not allowing them to think in terms of building a car.

Chapter Five: Insuring America

[1] Marc Steinberg, "Working without a Net," *Families USA,* April 2004, p. 1; http://www.familiesusa.org/site/DocServer/Holes_2004_update.pdf?docID=3304

[2] Dr. Roman Leibzon, personal communication, June 2004.

[3] Past honors have gone to the ENT, geriatric, and nephrology departments. *U.S. News & World Report's* "Best Hospitals 2004" is available at: http://www.usnews.com/usnews/health/hosptl/tophosp.htm

[4] Hillary Rodham Clinton, "Now Can We Talk about Health Care?" *New York Times Magazine,* April 18, 2004, p. 26.

[5] Matthew Miller, *The Two Percent Solution: Fixing America's Problems in Ways Liberals and Conservatives Can Love* (New York: PublicAffairs Books, 2003), pp. 112–13.

[6] Milt Freudenheim, "Record Level of Americans Not Insured on Health," *New York Times,* August 27, 2004.

[7] Douglas Holtz-Eakin, "Health Care Spending and the Uninsured," Testimony before the U.S. Senate Committee on Health, Education, Labor, and Pensions, January 28, 2004; http://www.cbo.gov/showdoc.cfm?index=4989&sequence=0

[8] My colleague, Dr. Shapasnikov, had a particularly telling story: "There have been times when I work up a patient, and then I call in the family for the bad news. Everyone sits around the table. I hold the patient's hand and say, 'you have cancer.' They then nod and say that they know, their doctor in Mexico already told them."

[9] The CPS does an annual survey, asking people if they were insured for the last calendar year, excluding the past two months. Thus, people must calculate back fourteen months and ignore their present circumstance.

[10] "How Many People Lack Health Insurance and for How Long?" Congressional Budget Office, Washington, D.C., May 2003.

[11] David Henderson, "Myths about U.S. Health Care," in *Better Medicine: Reforming Canadian Health Care,* ed. David Gratzer (Montreal: ECW Press, 2002), pp. 177–78.

[12] Shailesh Bhandari and Robert Mills, "Dynamics of Economic Well Being: Health Insurance 1996–1999," U.S. Census Bureau, August 2003, p. 10.

[13] "How Many People Lack Health Insurance and for How Long?"

[14] "The Uninsured in America," BlueCross BlueShield Association, February 27, 2003; http://bcbshealthissues.com/relatives/20464.pdf

[15] J. M. Yegian, D. G. Pockell, M. D. Smith, and E. K. Murray, "The Nonpoor Uninsured in California, 1998,"*Health Affairs,* vol. 19, no. 4 (July/August 2000), pp. 171–77.

[16] Yegian et al. also calculate the average for this group: $1,083. They note: "The difference between the two values indicates that although most of the uninsured are obtaining relatively few services at a relatively low cost, a small proportion are high users with a heavy associated financial burden."

[17] Jack Hadley and John Holahan, "How Much Medical Care Do the Uninsured Use, and Who Pays For It?" *Health Affairs,* Web exclusive, February 12, 2003, p. 78; http://content.healthaffairs.org/cgi/content/full/hlthaff.w3.66v1/DC1

[18] They used the MAPS survey data, rather than CPS. Ibid.

[19] Hadley and Holahan also distinguish between those who go without insurance for a full year, and those who are uninsured for only part of the year. The fully uninsured spend less, at $1,253, compared with $1,950 for the latter. Ibid.

[20] Ibid.

21 "IOM Report Calls for Universal Health Coverage by 2010; Offers Principles to Judge, Compare Proposed Solutions," Institute of Medicine press release, January 14, 2004.

22 Institute of Medicine, *Insuring America's Health: Principles and Recommendations* (Washington, D.C.: National Academies Press, 2004), p. 18.

23 David Frum, "Health Care: Beware the 'Little Fix,'" *Weekly Standard,* January 13, 1997; http://www.davidfrum.com/archive.asp?YEAR=1997

24 Paul Starr, "What Happened to Health Care Reform?" *American Prospect,* vol. 6, no. 20 (December 1, 1995); http://www.prospect.org/print/V6/20/starr-p.html

25 John McClaughry, personal communication, January 6, 2004.

26 Victoria Craig Bunce, personal communication, January 2004.

27 As quoted in: Conrad F. Meier, "Health Insurance Meltdown in Vermont," *Health Care News,* March 1, 2004; http://www.heartland.org/Article.cfm?artId=14530

28 The Vermont state government provides information on all registered companies. See: http://www.bishca.state.vt.us/HcaDiv/consumerpubs_healthcare/Shop_Indiv_SmallGroup/carriersindiv.htm

29 The following state summaries are based on: Victoria Craig Bunce, "What Were These States Thinking? The Pitfalls of Guaranteed Issue," *Issues & Answers,* no. 104, Council for Affordable Health Insurance, May 2002.

30 Victoria Craig Bunce and J. P. Wieske, "Health Insurance Mandates in the States, 2004," Council for Affordable Health Insurance, Alexandria, Virginia, 2004.

31 "The Cost and Benefits of Individual Health Insurance Plans," eHealthInsurance, September 2004; http://image.ehealthinsurance.com/ehealthinsurance/pressNew/ReportLink.html

32 "The Most Affordable Cities for Family Health Insurance," eHealthInsurance, December 7, 2004; http://image.ehealthinsurance.com/ehealthinsurance/pressNew/ReportLink.html

33 RAND Health, "State Efforts to Insure the Uninsured: The Unfinished Story," July 2004; http://www.rand.org/pubs/research_briefs/RB4558-1/index1.html

34 Martin Feldstein, "Health and Taxes," *Wall Street Journal,* January 19, 2004.

35 Shadegg's Health Care Choice Act is not perfect. First, he limits out-of-state purchases to individuals. Small businesses, however, would benefit as well from a stronger marketplace. Second, he allows premium taxes to be collected by the state where the individual resides, rather than the state of purchase. Looking to banking reforms, it seems that

allowing the premium tax to stay in the state of purchase would encourage some states to become hubs of insurance and regulatory enforcement.

[36] John F. Cogan, R. Glenn Hubbard, and Daniel P. Kessler, "Brilliant Deduction," *Wall Street Journal,* December 8, 2004. They also suggest allowing all out-of-pocket expenditures to be given tax preference.

Chapter Six: Mills' Revenge: Medicaid

[1] Martin Gottlieb, "A Managed Care Cure—All with Flaws and Potential," *New York Times,* October 1, 1995, p. A1. Martin Gottlieb, "A Free-for-All in Swapping Medicaid for Managed Care," *New York Times,* October 1, 1995, p. A1.

[2] G. Gordon Bonnyman Jr., "Stealth Reform: Market-Based Medicaid in Tennessee," *Health Affairs,* vol. 15, no. 2 (Summer 1996), p. 310.

[3] John K. Iglehart, "Medicaid," *New England Journal of Medicine,* vol. 340, no. 5 (February 4, 1999), p. 403.

[4] Ibid.

[5] Congressional Budget Office, "The Budget and Economic Outlook: Fiscal Years 2006 to 2015," Washington, D.C., January 2005; http://www.cbo.gov/showdoc.cfm?index=1821&sequence=0&from=7#t5

[6] The federal-state idea was borrowed from the Medicare proposals floated in the early 1960s by conservative legislators.

[7] The Federal Medical Assistance Percentage (FMAP) is the formula used to calculate the federal contribution to each state's program. Today, wealthier states, like New York and California, receive 50 cents on the Medicaid dollar from federal coffers; relatively poor states like Mississippi get more, as much as 76 cents (and, historically, even more). Overall, roughly 57% of Medicaid's budget is from Washington.

[8] When this proposal fell through, the Reagan administration attempted in 1982 to do a swap: the federal government would take over Medicaid and leave welfare to the individual states. This idea, too, fell through.

[9] Governor Bill Owens, personal communication, August 1, 2005.

[10] "HillaryCare in Tennessee," *Wall Street Journal,* December 6, 2004; http://www.opinionjournal.com/editorial/feature.html?id=110005987

[11] Christopher J. Conover, "Effects of Tennessee Medicaid Managed Care on Obstetrical Care and Birth Outcomes," *Journal of Health Politics, Policy and Law,* vol. 26, no. 6 (December 2001), pp. 1291–324.

[12] Notes Conover et al. in the introduction: "There is evidence that TennCare has increased use of preventive services, including immunization,

well-child visits, and mammograms and Pap smears. TennCare is also associated with reductions in emergency visits and hospital admissions for asthma patients. On the other hand, there is evidence of lower levels of prenatal care, obstetrical services, and physician-attended births. The percentage of low-income people making dental visits has also declined.... [T]here is mixed evidence on TennCare's effect on morbidity and mortality." See: Christopher J. Conover and Hester J. Davies, "The Role of TennCare in Health Policy for Low-Income People in Tennessee," Occasional Paper no. 33, The Urban Institute, Washington, D.C., 2000.

13 Michael Virtanen, "New York Audit: Sex Offenders Getting Viagra," Associated Press, May 22, 2005. Even the *New York Times* acknowledges that Medicaid "has been misspending billions of dollars annually because of fraud, waste and profiteering." See: Clifford J. Levy and Michael Luo, "Medicaid Fraud May Reach into Billions," *New York Times,* July 18, 2005, p. A1.

14 John K. Iglehart, "The Dilemma of Medicaid," *New England Journal of Medicine,* vol. 348, no. 21 (May 22, 2003).

15 Based on figures from the House Committee on Ways and Means, 2004 Green Book, 15-13; http://waysandmeans.house.gov/Documents.asp?section=813

16 "White House Rankled by Rice Delay," CBS.com, January 20, 2005; http://kutv.com/topstories/topstories_story_020110435.html

17 Robert Pear, "Bush Nominee Wants States to Get Medicaid Flexibility," *New York Times,* January 19, 2005.

18 Pam Belluck, "Governors Unite in Fight against Medicaid Cuts," *New York Times,* December 26, 2004.

19 Mark Duggan, "Does Contracting Out Increase the Efficiency of Government Programs? Evidence from Medicaid HMOs," NBER Working Paper no. 9091, August 2002, p. 10.

20 Ibid.

21 Based on a survey of pediatricians. Iglehart, "The Dilemma of Medicaid," p. 2144.

22 The survey also suggests that roughly one-third of American physicians decline all Medicaid patients. See: J. A. Schoenman and J. Feldman, *Results of the Medicare Payment Advisory Commission's 2002 Survey of Physicians* (Washington, D.C.: MedPac, 2003).

23 Governor Jeb Bush, "Medicaid Today: The States' Perspective," Hearings of the House Subcommittee on Health, March 12, 2003; http://energycommerce.house.gov/108/Hearings/03122003hearing815/Bush1332.htm

[24] Mark Duggan and Fiona Scott Morton, "The Distortionary Effects of Government Procurement: Evidence from Medicaid Prescription Drug Purchasing," NBER Working Paper no. W10980, December 2004.

[25] Based on data from the National Conference of State Legislatures. See: http://www.ncsl.org/programs/health/medicaidrx.htm

[26] Jim Frogue, personal communication, February 3, 2005.

[27] Peter J. Cunningham, "Medicaid Cost Containment and Access to Prescription Drugs," *Health Affairs,* vol. 24, no. 3 (May/June 2005), p. 788.

[28] Jay Bhattacharya, Dana Goldman, and Neeraj Sood, "The Link between Public and Private Insurance and HIV-Related Mortality," NBER Working Paper no. 9346, November 2002, p. 1.

[29] Sarah Lueck, "Creative Accounting for Medicaid," *Wall Street Journal,* February 24, 2005, p. A4.

[30] Ibid.

[31] Jonathan Weisman, "Medicaid Accounting Tactic Is Criticized by Lawmakers," *Washington Post,* April 8, 2005, p. A23.

[32] Michael Cannon at the Cato Institute has written well on this topic. See, for example: "Welfare Reform's Unfinished Business," *National Review Online,* May 17, 2005; http://www.nationalreview.com/comment/ cannon200505170805.asp

[33] More recently, RAND senior economists Stephen H. Long and M. Susan Marquis looked at seven states that expanded coverage for Medicaid between 1991 and 1997. They found that Medicaid enrollment increased—but private insurance enrollment also dropped. "About 50 percent of those who newly participated in the public program substituted public insurance for private insurance." See: "State Efforts to Insure the Uninsured: An Unfinished Story," RAND Health, http://www.rand.org/publications/RB/RB4558-1/

[34] President Clinton never embraced block grants, but—recognizing the problems of the present system—he suggested that Washington cap its future contributions.

[35] Jim Frogue, personal communication, February 3, 2005.

[36] The 2006 budget didn't include the proposal, either.

[37] Robert Pear, "States Propose Sweeping Changes to Trim Medicaid by Billions," *New York Times,* May 9, 2005; http://www.nytimes.com/2005/05/09/national/09medicaid.html

[38] Governor Mark Sanford, "Escaping the Morass: South Carolina's Plan to Transform Medicaid," Address to the Heritage Foundation, February 28, 2005.

[39] For a more detailed explanation, see: "Medicaid for Millionaires," *Wall Street Journal,* February 24, 2005.

[40] Ibid.

[41] "The Interaction of Public and Private Insurance: Medicaid and the Long-Term Care Insurance Market," NBER Working Paper no. 10989, December 2004.

[42] Several legislators in Ohio, for example, floated the idea of the state claiming a senior's assets, then offering him or her a no-interest loan. Once the senior dies, the state would offset Medicaid costs against the assets.

[43] Michael Bond, personal communication, April 2005.

[44] Jim Frogue, "Medicaid's Perverse Incentives," American Legislative Exchange Council, Washington, D.C., July 2004, p. 6.

[45] Governor Bill Owens, personal communication, August 1, 2005.

[46] John Andrews, "Rocky Mountain Medicaid," Wall Street Journal, August 18, 2005, p. A1.

Chapter Seven: Mills' Revenge II: Medicare

[1] Tom DeLay, "Medicare Reform," Washington Times, November 20, 2003; http://www.washingtontimes.com/op-ed/20031120-075900-7874r.htm

[2] For example, former Speaker of the House Newt Gingrich suggested that "if you are a fiscal conservative . . . there may be no more important a vote in your career than one in support of this bill." See: Newt Gingrich, "Conservatives Should Vote 'Yes' on Medicare," Wall Street Journal, November 20, 2003.

[3] Sally Pipes, "Costly Prescriptions," National Review Online, November 19, 2003; http://www.nationalreview.com/comment/pipes 200311191033.asp

[4] Dick Armey, "Vote 'No' to the Medicare Bill," Wall Street Journal, November 21, 2003.

[5] The structure is as follows: after meeting a $250 deductible, insurance will pay 75% of drug costs up to $2,250, but then there will be no coverage for drugs between $2,250 and $3,600. Over $3,600, there will be 95% coverage.

[6] Milton Friedman, personal communication, November 8, 2003.

[7] Michael L. Gillette, "Wilbur Mills Oral History, Interview II," LBJ Library, March 25, 1987; http://www.ssa.gov/history/pdf/mills2.pdf

[8] "2005 Annual Report of the Boards of Trustees of the Federal Hospital Insurance and Federal Supplementary Medical Insurance Trust Funds," p. 23; http://www.cms.hhs.gov/publications/trusteesreport/ tr2005.pdf

[9] Reischauer has made these comments on several occasions; see for example the Urban Institute roundtable discussion of January 5, 1999; http://www.urban.org/url.cfm?ID=900312

[10] Gina Kolata, "Patients in Florida Lining Up for All That Medicare Covers," *New York Times,* September 13, 2003, p. A1.

[11] John E. Wennberg, Elliott S. Fisher, Therese A. Stukel, and Sandra M. Sharp, "Use of Medicare Claims Data to Monitor Provider-Specific Performance among Patients with Severe Chronic Illness," *Health Affairs,* Web exclusive, October 7, 2004; http://content.healthaffairs.org/cgi/content/abstract/hlthaff.var.5v1

[12] Elliott S. Fisher, David E. Wennberg, Therese A. Stukel, and Daniel J. Gottlieb, "Variations in the Longitudinal Efficiency of Academic Medical Centers," *Health Affairs,* Web exclusive, October 7, 2004; http://content.healthaffairs.org/cgi/content/abstract/hlthaff.var.19

[13] Jonathan Skinner, Elliott S. Fisher, and John E. Wennberg, "The Efficiency of Medicare," NBER Working Paper no. 8395, July 2001.

[14] Gilbert M. Gaul, "Bad Practices Net Hospitals More Money: High Quality Often Loses Out in the 40-Year-Old Program," *Washington Post,* July 24, 2005, p. A1.

[15] Centers for Medicare & Medicaid Services, "Medicare Estimated Benefit Payments by State, Fiscal Year 2001," Baltimore, September 2002; http://cms.hhs.gov/statistics/feeforservice/BenefitPayments01

[16] Laurie McGinley and Sarah Lueck, "As the Medicare Chief Reins in Costs, Opposition Grows: Drug, Device Makers Rue Scully's Decisions," *Wall Street Journal,* July 16, 2003, p. A1.

[17] Ibid.

[18] Matthew Miller, *The Two Percent Solution: Fixing America's Problems in Ways Liberals and Conservatives Can Love* (New York: PublicAffairs Books, 2003), p. 209.

[19] Peter J. Cunningham, Andrea Staiti, and Paul B. Ginsburg, "Physician Acceptance of New Medicare Patients Stabilizes in 2004–05," Tracking Report no. 12, Center for Studying Health System Change, January 2006; http://hschange.org/CONTENT/811/?topic=topic16

[20] As cited in: Kathleen Murray, Testimony of the American Hospital Association before the Task Force on Health of the Budget Committee, U.S. House of Representatives, "Complexity and Burden of Medicare Regulations on Providers," May 18, 2000; http://www.aha.org/aha/advocacy-grassroots/advocacy/

[21] American Hospital Association, "Patients or Paperwork? The Regulatory Burden Facing America's Hospitals," 2001; http://www.aha.org/aha/advocacy-grassroots/

[22] Federal Trade Commission and Department of Justice, *Improving Health Care: A Dose of Competition,* Washington, D.C., July 2004, p. 9; http://www.ftc.gov/opa/2004/07/healthcarerpt.htm

23 Uwe E. Reinhardt, "The Medicare World from Both Sides: A Conversation with Tom Scully," *Health Affairs,* vol. 22, no. 6 (November/December 2003), p. 168.

24 Robert E. Moffit, "A Road Map for Medicare Reform: Building on the Experience of the FEHBP," Testimony before the Senate Special Committee on Aging, May 6, 2003; http://aging.senate.gov/public/_files/hr99rm.pdf

25 Harry P. Cain, "Moving Medicare to the FEHBP Model, or How to Make an Elephant Fly: Can Medicare Really Be Modernized?" *Health Affairs,* vol. 18, no. 4 (July/August 1999), p. 26.

26 The federal government contribution is equal to the lesser of: (1) 72% of the program-wide weighted average of premiums, or (2) 75% of the total for the particular plan an enrollee selects.

27 Walton Francis, *Checkbook's Guide to Health Plans for Federal Employees* (Washington, D.C.: Washington Center for the Study of Services, 2002), p. 80.

28 For an eloquent comparison of the FEHBP and Medicare, particularly with regard to cost control, see: Joseph P. Antos, "The Role of Market Competition in Strengthening Medicare," Testimony before the Senate Special Committee on Aging, May 6, 2003.

29 Cain, "Moving Medicare to the FEHBP Model," p. 30.

30 Joint Economic Committee, U.S. Congress: http://jec.senate.gov/_files/HealthInsuranceGrowth.pdf

31 Obviously, Medicare doesn't treat everyone perfectly equally. Some poorer elderly, for example, have historically qualified for Medicaid. As well, with the Medicare Modernization Act of 2003, there is some modest differential in terms of fees.

32 Part D does, however, offer subsidies to lower-income seniors.

Chapter Eight: Our Drug Problem

1 Richard Epstein, "Regulatory Paternalism in the Market for Drugs: Lessons from Vioxx and Celebrex," *Yale Journal of Health Policy, Law, and Ethics,* vol. 2 (2005), p. 106.

2 The otherwise sober *Lancet* editorialized: "Drug regulators must now reassess the safety and efficacy thresholds required for the licensing of a new pharmaceutical product.... Without more vigilant drug regulation in the future, doctors will continue to be misled and patients' lives will continue to be endangered." See: "Vioxx: An Unequal Partnership between Safety and Efficacy," *Lancet,* vol. 364, no. 9442 (October 2000), p. 1287.

3 "It's Not about the Bike, It's about Clinical Trials," IU Home Pages, October 3, 2003; http://www.homepages.indiana.edu/100303/text/armstrongteam.shtml

[4] "Views on Prescription Drugs and the Pharmaceutical Industry," Kaiser Health Poll Report, January/February 2005; http://www.kff.org/healthpollreport/feb_2005/index.cfm

[5] As quoted in: Joe Moser, "Drug Reimportation Measure Passes House," *Health Care News,* September 1, 2003; http://www.heartland.org/ Article.cfm?artId=12764

[6] Rep. Gil Gutknecht (R-Minn.) championed the idea when I debated him in a panel discussion at the American Enterprise Institute on October 2, 2003.

[7] "Cancer Prognosis," *Wall Street Journal,* February 26, 2006; based on National Center for Health Statistics.

[8] Gardiner Harris, "Prilosec's Maker Switches Users to Nexium, Thwarting Generics," *Wall Street Journal,* June 6, 2002, p. A1.

[9] Merrill Goozner, *The $800 Million Pill: The Truth Behind the Costs of New Drugs* (Los Angeles: University of California Press, 2004), p. 222.

[10] Jalpa A. Doshi, Nicole Brandt, and Bruce Stuart, "The Impact of Drug Coverage on COX-2 Inhibitor Use in Medicare," *Health Affairs,* Web exclusive, February 18, 2004, pp. 94–105, quoted at 102; http://content.healthaffairs.org/cgi/content/full/hlthaff.w4.94v1?

[11] John Goodman, personal communication, June 22, 2005, based on Aetna Health Fund data.

[12] Dr. Henry Miller, personal communication, November 6, 2003.

[13] Scott Gottlieb, "The Great Shift to Specialty Drugs," On the Issues, American Enterprise Institute, June 2005; http://www.aei.org/publications/ pubID.22748.filter.all/pub_detail.asp

[14] Sam Kazman, "Deadly Overcaution: FDA's Drug Approval Process," *Journal of Regulation and Social Costs,* vol. 1 (August 1990), pp. 42–43.

[15] Kazman actually does estimate the number—twenty to fifty thousand lives.

[16] As quoted in Daniel P. Carpenter, "The Political Economy of FDA Drug Review: Processing, Politics, and Lessons for Policy," *Health Affairs,* vol. 23, no. 1 (January/February 2004), p. 54. Former FDA general counsel Peter Barton Hutt has echoed Schmidt: "FDA employees have been praised only for refusing to approve a new drug, not for making a courageous judgment to approve a new drug that has in fact helped patients and advanced the public health." As quoted in Henry Miller, "The Curse of Too Much Caution," *Wall Street Journal,* November 26, 2004.

[17] "Pazdur's Cancer Rules," *Wall Street Journal,* July 6, 2005, p. A14.

[18] Scott Gottlieb, "Opening Pandora's Pillbox: Using Modern Information Tools to Improve Drug Safety," *Health Affairs,* vol. 24, no. 4 (July/August 2005).

[19] Miller, "The Curse of Too Much Caution."

[20] Gottlieb, "Opening Pandora's Pillbox," p. 939.

[21] As compared with just 20,455 from individuals and physicians. Ibid., p. 941.

[22] Ibid., p. 944.

Chapter Nine: The Hip That Changed History

[1] Dr. Brian Day, personal communication, March 3, 2006. I wrote more detailed comments about the interview in "The Hip That Changed Health Care History," *National Past* (Canada), March 7, 2006.

[2] Bill Virgin, "Health Insurance System Hangs On," *Seattle Post-Intelligencer,* November 12, 2002

[3] Ceci Connolly and Amy Goldstein, "Health Insurance Back As Key Issue," *Washington Post,* March 16, 2003, p. A5.

[4] Ibid.

[5] The two women were featured in a Canadian Broadcasting Corporation special. See: http://www.cbc.ca/webone/borderlinehealthcare/hcg_main.swf. In addition, personal communications with Donna Longmoore and Christina Alcorn, January 5, 2003.

[6] Some basic health services, though, are not—dentistry, crutches for a broken leg, eye examinations.

[7] Ipsos-Reid Media Release, "Healthcare in Canada: Eight in Ten (78%) of Canadians Agree That the Healthcare System in Their Province Is Currently in a Crisis," February 2, 2000.

[8] Standing Senate Committee on Social Affairs, Science and Technology, *The Health of Canadians—The Federal Role,* vol. 5, *Principles and Recommendations for Reform—Part I* (Ottawa, April 2002). Such stories are commonly reported: "The Long, Long Wait in Great Pain: From Being Put on List for Hip Replacement to Operation May Take 15 Months," *Montreal Gazette;* "'Patients Deserve Better,' Fed-Up Canadian Says," *Edmonton Journal;* "Heart-Surgery Wait Claims 3 Lives: 47 More Patients Languishing on List," *Winnipeg Free Press;* "Provinces Spend Millions on U.S. Care for Patients," *Globe and Mail.*

[9] Nadeem Esmail and Michael Walker, *Waiting Your Turn: Hospital Waiting Lists in Canada,* 15th ed. (Vancouver, B.C.: The Fraser Institute, 2005).

[10] Stories abound: when a hospital tried to give away one of its ultrasound machines to a local vet, he declined—he had better equipment. Concerned about medico-legal implications, the Canadian Association of Radiologists commissioned a legal opinion. Lawyers advised our radiologists to tell patients to "shop around" for facilities with

newer equipment—even if it means looking outside Canada, since "[I]t is imperative that the patient ... understand the risks and uncertainties associated with the reliability of such ... examination[s]." See: Canadian Association of Radiologists, *Special Ministerial Briefing— Outdated Radiology Equipment: A Diagnostic Crisis* (Saint-Laurent, Quebec: September 2000), p. 7.

[11] Researchers attributed the difference partly to the availability of angioplasty and bypass surgery north and south of the 49th parallel. "No question, [Americans] are more aggressive in the early management of heart attacks," observes Dr. Anthony Graham, a Toronto cardiologist. See: Brad Evenson, "Cardiac Care Better in U.S., Study Shows: Fewer Are Dying, but Canadian Heart Attack Patients Have Poorer Quality of Life," *National Post,* February 8, 2001, p. A4.

[12] For a more extensive discussion, please see: David Gratzer, ed., *Better Medicine: Reforming Canadian Health Care* (Montreal: ECW Press, 2002).

[13] A paper in *Health Affairs* opens: "Americans have often looked with envy at the German health care system where citizens enjoy universal access to a comprehensive set of health benefits, all for about half of what Americans pay per capita. As if that weren't enough, outcomes and satisfaction in Germany are at least as good as (if not better than) those in the United States." See: Alison Evans Cuellar and Joshua M. Wiener, "Can Social Insurance for Long Term Care Work? The Experience of Germany," *Health Affairs,* vol. 19, no. 3 (May/June 2000), p. 8. The editors of journals aren't the only ones with a keen interest in Europe; Howard Dean, when governor of Vermont, saw the continent's social insurances as the inspiration for his health reforms.

[14] Almost one-third of patients face no user fee at all, while the majority pay just a fraction of even the smallest of medical bills. Family physicians, thus, spend part of their day entertaining the bored elderly— and prescribing them medications. French patients are prescribed more drugs than their counterparts anywhere else. How to provide so much for so many? France underpays physicians, blocks new (and expensive) drugs from reaching patients, and limits the number of medical graduates.

[15] Philippe Manière, "Perspectives on European Health Care," Lecture at the Heritage Foundation, Washington, D.C., April 26, 2001.

[16] Cathy Schoen, Robert J. Blendon, Catherine M. DesRoches, and Robin Osborn, "Comparison of Health Care System Views and Experiences in Five Nations, 2001," Commonwealth Fund, Issue Brief, May 2002.

[17] Gerard F. Anderson, Uwe E. Reinhardt, Peter S. Hussey, and Varduhi Petrosyan, "It's the Prices, Stupid: Why the United States Is So Different

from Other Countries," *Health Affairs,* vol. 22, no. 3 (May/June 2003), Exhibit 5.

18 Axel Morer-Funk, "The German Health Care System: Facts, Problems, and Reform Proposals," Goethe-Institut Inter Nationes, 2002.

19 W. Allen Wallis, *An Overgoverned Society* (New York: Free Press, 1976), p. 256.

20 Milton Friedman, "How to Cure Health Care," *Public Interest,* Winter 2001, p. 32.

21 David Harriman, William McArthur, and Martin Zelder, *The Availability of Medical Technology in Canada: An International Comparative Study,* Public Policy Sources no. 20 (Vancouver, B.C.: Fraser Institute, 1999).

22 Paul Krugman, "Ailing Health Care," *New York Times,* April 11, 2005, p. A19.

23 J. E. Becerra, C. J. Hogue, H. K. Atrash, and N. Pérez, "Infant Mortality among Hispanics: A Portrait of Heterogeneity," *Journal of the American Medical Association,* vol. 265, no. 2 (January 9, 1991), pp. 217–21.

24 Paul Krugman, "The Medical Money Pit," *New York Times,* April 15, 2005, p. A19.

25 "The U.S. takes an aggressive approach towards early screening, early diagnosis and early treatment of breast cancer," notes Datamonitor's cancer analyst Richard Andrews. "They have left other nations far behind and this strategy is reflected in the U.S. having the best 5 year survivals for breast cancer, more than any other country." Indeed, in the United States, women age forty and over are advised to get yearly mammograms. In the United Kingdom, in contrast, women are told to wait until age fifty—and then to get the test only every three years. See: Richard Woodman, "Breast Cancer Diagnosed Late in Europe," Reuters Health, March 3, 2003.

26 Global Action Against Cancer, World Health Organization, Geneva, Switzerland, 2003; http://www.uicc.org/index.php?id=497

27 Gerard F. Anderson and Peter S. Hussey, "Multinational Comparisons of Health Systems Data," Commonwealth Fund, October 2000.

28 Ibid.

29 Karen Donelan et al., "The Cost of Health System Change: Public Discontent in Five Nations," *Health Affairs,* May/June 1999.

30 Oliver Schöffski, "Diffusion of Medicines in Europe," prepared for the European Federation of Pharmaceutical Industries and Associations, December 2002; http://www.gm.wiso.uni-erlangen.de/

31 Treatment of another mental illness is surprisingly different in the United States and across the Atlantic. Antipsychotics, the main treat-

ment for schizophrenia, have been revolutionized in the past decade. Newer drugs are linked with fewer and more benign side effects. In the United States, 60% of patients are on the newer drugs. In Spain, only 20% are, and in Germany, fewer still—just 10%.

[32] In a recent paper, Prof. Patricia Danzon of the University of Pennsylvania finds that in regulation-heavy countries like Greece, Belgium, and France, medications take an extra nine months *after* EU approval to reach patients. Patricia M. Danzon, Y. Richard Wang, and Liang Wang, "The Impact of Price Regulation on the Launch Delay of New Drugs— A Study of Twenty-Five Major Markets in the 1990s," at Prof Danzon's website: http://hc.wharton.upenn.edu/danzon/ (The paper is under review by *Law & Economics.*)

[33] Borrowed from the *Wall Street Journal* editorial by this name.

[34] Department of Health, *A Concordat with the Private and Voluntary Health Care Provider Sector,* October 31, 2000, Introduction. In the words of Nick Mathiason of the *Observer,* "[The Concordat] smashed 50 years of ideological hostility towards private medicine." The *Financial Times* declared it the most important NHS document in five decades.

[35] Roughly one in five elective surgeries in Britain are performed in the non-NHS operating theaters, including heart bypasses and other "major" surgery. Adding up all the hospital and long-term beds provided by the independent sector yields a staggering number: 440,000 beds—more than the NHS and local authorities combined. The independent sector employs over three-quarters of a million people. Total care in private hands accounts for nearly 25 cents on every dollar of health and social-care spending in Britain.

[36] Greg Scandlen, "Australia Ends Community Rating," NCPA's *Health Policy Week* no. 169, June 3, 2001; based on Sharon Willcox, "Promoting Private Health Insurance in Australia," Market Watch, *Health Affairs,* May/June 2001.

[37] The data for the Stockholm Model draws from a chapter I co-authored with council adviser Johan Hjertqvist. For further details, please see this chapter: "Health Reform Abroad," in *Better Medicine: Reforming Canadian Health Care,* ed. David Gratzer (Montreal: ECW Press, 2002).

[38] Based on a blog by Tim Evans, president of the Centre for the New Europe, at: http://www.cnehealth.org

[39] Annette Tuffs, "Germany Expects More Hospital Privatization," *British Medical Journal,* vol. 320 (April 15, 2000), p. 1030.

[40] John Martin of the Organisation for Economic Co-operation and Development notes that the reforms "encourage better service and institute incentives for administrative cost reduction." See: "The Experience

of OECD Countries in Containing Rising Health Costs," Testimony
before the Joint Economic Committee, U.S. Congress, April 10, 2003.
[41] Ibid.

Chapter Ten: The Three Keys

[1] Susan Chambers, "Reviewing and Revising Wal-Mart's Benefits Strategy," Memorandum to the Board of Directors, p. 14. This confidential
memo is available on the *New York Times* website: http://www.nytimes.
com/packages/pdf/business/26walmart.pdf

[2] Andrew J. Rettenmaier and Thomas Saving, *The Economics of Medicare
Reform* (Kalamazoo, Michigan: W. E. Upjohn Institute for Employment
Research, 2000), p. 30.

[3] Milton Friedman, personal correspondence, November 24, 2004.

[4] Eduardo Porter, "Health Care for All, Just a (Big) Step Away," *New York
Times,* December 18, 2005.

[5] The health-tax exclusion, after all, has grown into a tax break for middle and high earners. From a tax policy perspective, this tax break
doesn't make much sense (thus my belief that it should be ended).
But to eliminate the deduction without a compensatory cut in taxes
would mean a heavy increase in taxes for millions of Americans. That's
not our aim: tax reform ought to be neutral. The purpose of this exercise is to improve American health care. Thus a sensible approach
would be to eliminate the deduction *and* cut taxes accordingly.

[6] Marc L. Berk and Alain C. Monheit, "The Concentration of Health Care
Expenditures, Revisited," *Health Affairs,* vol. 20, no. 2 (March/April
2001), pp. 9–18.

[7] There are ways to tackle the pooling issue, which may appeal to those
who favor market solutions yet aren't as libertarian as Prof. Friedman.
For instance, we could nationalize the pricing of health insurance. As
Prof. Regina Herzlinger (Harvard) points out, in Switzerland, people
pay for policies based on their age, with subsidies for lower-income
citizens. A 55-year-old gentleman in good health would then pay the
same as his neighbor who suffers from heart disease. Thus, cross-sub-
sidization would alleviate the burden of chronic illness. Even if risk-
pooling is a priority, holding on to the status quo isn't necessary. A
quasi-socialist, Swiss-style scheme, in which prices are regulated cen-
trally and pooled, would allow everyone affordable insurance (and
not strap us to a 1940s paradigm).

It should also be noted that objections to variation in premiums turn
on a principle—equity—that isn't applied in any other sector of the
economy. Should health insurance cost roughly the same amount to

everyone involved? Would we apply such a standard to food? Is it fair that some people have full meals with appetizers and desserts at higher costs, while others simply have lower-cost main courses? By focusing on equality (really the issue when people say that those of poorer health will be discriminated against by individual insurance pricing), we ignore the fact that people make a choice when deciding on insurance. After all, not all insurance is equal—and thus neither are premiums. People demanding comprehensive insurance, with minimal copays and deductibles, are undoubtedly going to have to pay more—in the way that people who opt for a gas-guzzling V6 will pay more at the pump than those who want a 4-cylinder hybrid.

[8] Alan Greenspan, Remarks to the Federal Reserve Bank of Philadelphia Policy Forum, December 2, 2005; http://federalreserve.gov/boarddocs/speeches/2005/20051202/default.htm

[9] To put it slightly differently, for every retiree, four workers pay tax. That number will drop to 2.4 by 2030.

[10] Quoted in Rettenmaier and Saving. *The Economics of Medicare Reform,* p. 32.

[11] Ibid.

[12] Alan Greenspan, Remarks to the Federal Reserve Bank of Philadelphia Policy Forum, December 2, 2005.

[13] Prof. Martin Feldstein (Harvard) estimated that depositing roughly 1.4% of total payroll into personal accounts would be sufficient. "In the long run, the accounts would eliminate the need for massive taxes that would otherwise reduce disposable income of low- and middle-income workers by 20% and impose an extra deadweight loss equal to more than six percent of existing wages." See: Martin Feldstein, "Prefunding Medicare," NBER Working Paper no. 6917, January 1999, p. 10. But years have passed since Prof. Feldstein made this calculation—which undercuts the potential gains of compound interest. More significantly, it makes limited sense to speculate exactly how much money would need to be placed in private accounts.

[14] Gary Becker, "Big Ideas," *Milken Institute Review,* 2nd qtr. (June) 2004, pp. 93–94; http://www.milkeninstitute.org/publications/review/2004_6/93_94mr22.pdf

[15] Sarah F. Jagger, "Prescription Drugs: Implications of Drug Labeling and Off-Label Use," Testimony before the Subcommittee on Human Resources and Intergovernmental Relations, U.S. House of Representatives, September 12, 1996.

Index

National Center for Health Statistics, 174

National Center for Policy Analysis, 62, 64, 123, 138, 147

National Coalition on Health Care, 163

National Governors' Conference, 46

Netherlands, 181

New England Journal of Medicine, 90

New Hampshire, 98

Newhouse, Joseph, 21, 70

New Jersey, 94, 96, 98, 99

New Republic, 163

New Statesman, 30

Newsweek, 15

New York, 98, 99; Medicaid in, 105–6

New York Presbyterian Hospital, 60

New York Times, 53, 68; on Medicare, 127; and tax exemption, 186; on TennCare, 101; on uninsured numbers, 82, 83

New Zealand, 171, 176–77

Nexium, 146, 148

Nixon, Richard, 6, 107; and HMOs, 45–46, 47, 57, 132

Nordhaus, William, 202

Observer, 33

Office of Management and Budget, 99, 189

Ohio, 96, 117, 163, 213

Oregon, 46, 129, 174; Measure 23, 162–63, 165

Organisation for Economic Co-operation and Development, 182

Osler, Sir William, 12, 14

Overgoverned Society, A (Wallis), 173

Owens, Bill, 104, 119

Palm Beach Gardens Medical Center, 128

Pataki, George, 105

Patient Power (Goodman/Musgrave), 63

Pawlecki, Brent, 41

penicillin, vii, 5, 13–14, 25, 29, 197

Pennsylvania, 110

PET (positron emission tomography) scans, 15

pharmaceutical industry: adverse reaction reports, 158; advertising, 41–42; drug withdrawals, 141–42, 151, 157, 158; litigation against, 158, 159; public opinion of, 143

pharmaceuticals, 8, 9, 14, 105; adverse effects, 154, 157–59; amoxicillin, 195; antipsychotics, 15, 193, 196; Avastin, 144–45; bromfenac, 157; in Canada, 143–44; for cancer, 142, 144–45, 151–52, 153, 178, 195; cardiac, 20; Claritin, 55; clozapine, 193; cost, 142, 147; for depression, 178; development expense, 152, 157–58; and electronic records, 158–59; Erbitux, 152; in Europe, 154, 160, 178; and FEHBP, 133–34; generics, 113, 145, 147, 148; and Internet pharmacies, 55, 71; Iressa, 151–52, 153; Marquibo, 152; and Medicaid regulations, 108–9; and Medicare, 121–24, 133–34, 137; Mevacor, 55; misoprostol, 150; naproxen, 147; Nexium, 146, 148; NSAIDs, 141, 147–48; off-label use, 152, 195; olanzapine, 193; over-the-counter sale, 55; Plan B (contraceptive), 151; Prilosec, 55; Prozac, 14, 178; reimportation, 142, 143–44; Rezulin, 151, 158; risperidone, 193; "self-prescribing" of, 55–56; SSRIs, 178; statins, 22; testing of, 154–58; U.S. innovation, 144–45,